KAVA-KAVA

Sacred Brew

by E. F. Steinmetz, Sc.D.

Derivative by Beverly A. Potter, Ph.D.

RONIN

Berkeley, California

KAVA-KAVA

Sacred Brew

by E. F. Steinmetz, Sc.D.

Derivative by Beverly A. Potter, Ph.D.

Kava Kava: Sacred Brew

Copyright: Ronin Publishing, 2017
ISBN: 9781579512316

Published by
RONIN Publishing, Inc.
PO Box 3436
Oakland CA 94609
www.roninpub.com

Production:
    Derivative Author: Beverly A. Potter, Ph.D.
    Book & Cover Design: Beverly A. Potter, Ph.D.
    Copy Editor: Mike Marinacci
    Photos: Fotolia

Library of Congress Card Number: 2017902697
Manufactured in the United States by Lightning Source.
Distributed to the book trade by PGW.

About the Author:

Dr. E. F. Steinmetz (1901-1972) was a Dutch botanist and the publisher-editor of *The Quarterly Journal of Crude Drug Research* and *Acto Phytotherapeutica*, as well as the author of several botanical lexicons, including *Codex Vegetabilis*, which includes names of drugs in several languages, and *Vocabularium Botanicum*, in Latin, Greek, Dutch, German, English and French, for which he was awarded the degree Ph.J. with *honoris causa*. He also authored *Drug Guide*, *Materia Medica Vegetabilis*, and *Piper Methysticum*—translates *Kava Root*.

As a young man, Dr. Steinmetz went to the far East, spending many years at Colombo (Ceylon), Medan (Sumatra), and Bandung (Java), returning to Holland shortly before World War II. He gained his great respect for the "natural" drugs from his experiences in the Asiatic world and often mentioned his remarkable observations made in Asia.

At 50 years old, he succumbed to poliomyelitis, which lead to being hospitalized two years, where he passed his time in studying botany and plant drugs. On December 25, 1972, Dr. Steinmetz passed away in Amsterdam, his natal city.

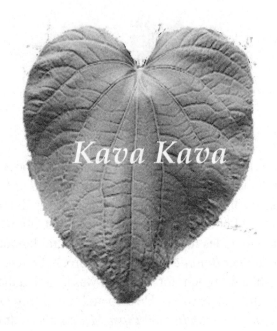

Kava Kava

Important Notice:

Information in this book is provided under the First Amendment of the Constitution and is not medical advice. Readers should discuss issues raised in this book with their personal physician and follow their physician's advice regarding it. Readers should also consult an attorney as to the legal status of kava-kava in their state and city.

Table of Contents

1. What is Kava Kava? 9
2. Kavalactones 14
3. Kava, the Plant 21
4. Kava Chemistry..................................29
5. Kava Root.......................................42
6. Effects of Kava Drinking 47
7. The Kava Brew 54
8. Preparing Brew at Home.........................62
9. Kava Bars.......................................70
10. Kava Therapeutics 77
11. Soothing Anxiety...............................83
12. Kava and Sleep.................................95
13. Don't Use Kava With Drugs.....................99
14. Liver Toxicity Risk 104
15. Bibliography 109
16. About Derivative Author......................115
17. Ronin Books-for-Independent-Minds...........117

What is Kava Kava?

Kava kava—*Piper methysticum*—is a tropical shrub that grows throughout the Pacific Islands. Kava kava belongs to the pepper family—*Piperaceae*—and is also known as kava, asava pepper, or intoxicating pepper. The root has been used as a medicine and in ceremonies for centuries.

The root and stems are made into a non-alcoholic, psychoactive beverage that has been used socially and ceremonially for hundreds of years in Hawaii, Fiji, and Tonga. Kava has a calming effect, producing brain wave changes similar to changes that occur with calming medicines such as Valium. Kava can prevent convulsions and relax muscles. Although kava is not addictive, it is habit-forming, while its effect tends to decrease with use. Kava root is available as a dietary supplement in powder and tincture forms.

> *Kava Kava is known as the intoxicating pepper.*

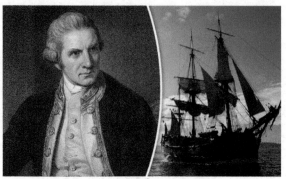
Captain J. Cook, 1728-1779

Long History

Drinking kava traces back at least 3,000 years and is associated with social and ceremonial functions. Captain James Cook, who discovered the South Pacific islands, was the first European to drink the kava brew and experience the preparation ritual.

When he discovered the island of Tonga in 1773, Cook noted in his journal that the Islanders came out in canoes to their ship to gave them kava root. Impressed by the gesture, Cook wrote: "One would not wish for a better sign of friendship than this; can we make a friend more welcome than by setting before him the best liquor in our possession?"

> *Captain James Cook was a British explorer, navigator, cartographer, and captain in the Royal Navy. Cook sailed thousands of miles in three voyages across uncharted areas of the globe. Cook mapped lands from New Zealand to Hawaii in the Pacific Ocean. Cook was attacked and killed in a confrontation with Hawaiians during his third exploratory voyage in the Pacific in 1779. Cook left a legacy of scientific and geographical knowledge.*

Daniel Carl Solander, a Swedish botanist and artist, Sydney Parkinson accompanied Captain *Cook* on his first voyage on the "Endeavour"

The Kava brew was used as a token of respect and goodwill, and is a ritual drink.

in 1768 and were charged with the important job of drawing the plants on the newly discovered islands. Johann Gearg Forster, who officially assigned kava its scientific name of *Piper methysticum*, accompanied Cook on his second voyage in 1772. Forster published the first notes on kava.

Cook's journal tells us that kava brew was widely used as a token of respect and goodwill. It was a ritual drink at magico-religious and ceremonial occasions.

Popular Drink

Kava's preparation has much ritual. The ground root and stems are placed into a porous sack, then submerged in a bowl of water, to be repeatedly squeezed into a large, carved, wooden bowl. When ready, coconut half-shell cups are dipped into the brew. After drinking there is a sense of heightened attention, as a wave of relaxation spreads. Kava brew is unlike alcohol because with kava, thoughts remain clear. The flavor is earthy and takes getting used to.

Drinking of kava is not confined to ceremonies. Kava is widely enjoyed, as we would drink

> *Kava brew is a habit-forming drink, and said to be irresistible once its taste is acquired.*

coffee and teas at home, with friends, and in the office. In the South Seas there is always a bowl of kava in the village as well as in many offices in the towns, and it is also drunk by most Indians and some Europeans in the South Pacific islands.

After Cook's discovery, European men in the Pacific took readily to kava drinking, for "its thirst-quenching and stimulating properties are unequaled". They reported that the taste was at first soapy, but soon changed into a pleasant feeling of freshness of the mouth, which lasted at least two hours. They said that the drink refreshed body and mind after long journeys, provided it is taken in moderate quantity.

When the White Man came to the Pacific islands, they plied the natives with liquor and taught them how to distill spirits. As these liquors were more potent than kava, the natives eagerly drank them, as they did with the comparatively harmless kava. Kava use decreased temporarily.

Nowadays the islanders drink a much weaker kava solution, though in larger quantities, and then mostly prepared by macerating the grated or pounded rootstock in cold water and coconut milk.

Steeped in Tradition

Cook's notes and those of subsequent explorers attested to kava's traditional central role in many ceremonies, including marriages, funerals, healing ceremonies, naming ceremonies, and initiation for young girls and boys.

> *It is obligatory to bring the kava root as a gift when visiting a new village.*

It is obligatory to bring the kava root as a gift when visiting a new village. The community then gathers to prepare the drink for communal drinking. After the village chief has his cup of kava, the drink is offered to the rest of the community in a communal bowl, which is passed around.

Etiquette is expected to be followed at a kava drinking party. Ignoring expected etiquette would be considered the height of ill-breeding. Before receiving the drink, tradition dictates clapping the hands once, then after finishing the drink, one has to clap three more times. When the ceremonial drinking is complete, everyone gathered has become friends, and the rest of the celebrations begin.

Kavalactones

The active ingredients in kava are phytochemicals called "kavalactones". Kavalactones give kava its stress-fighting, muscle-relaxing effects and are responsible for kava root's calming, anxiolytic, and euphoric effects.

Kavalactones are concentrated in the rootstock and roots not in the stems and leaves of the plant. There are eighteen types of kavalactones, but six of them represent greater than 90 percent of the total amount of kavalactones within the kava specimen. While each kavalactone produces a somewhat different physiologic effect in the body, a better effect is achieved when all work together than when any one kavalactone acts alone.

> KAVALACTONES *are a class of lactone compounds found in the roots of the kava shrub that have a variety of effects including amnestic, analgesic, anticonvulsant, anxiolytic, nootropic, and sedative/hypnotic experiences*

Calming Effect

German researcher Meyer found that the kava-lactones have a pronounced sedative effect, with the unsaturated kavalactones—kavain, methysticin, yangonin—more potent than the others.

Researchers Kretzschmar and Teschendor showed that the kavalactones do not induce sleep like an actual sedative but rather act as muscle relaxants and enhancers of deep sleep. Kavalactones appear to work on the limbic system of the brain.

Researchers Holm et al. showed that the kavalactone kavain increases the sensitivity of an area of the hippocampus, an area indirectly associated with emotional excitability due to its inhibition of the emotional centers of the brain cortex.

This agrees with kava drinkers' perceptions that kava has a calming effect. Kavalactones can act on the body in different ways

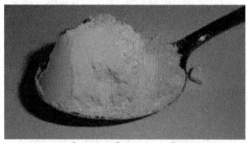

A moderate does is calming.

at different doses, which is part of what makes kava such a versatile calming herb: one suitable to help with daytime anxiety, evening recreation, and nighttime sleep alike.

Kavalactones Dosage

The kavalactones dosage in a traditionally prepared cold infusion of kava root can vary drastically, from 150 mg in a four-ounce serving to as much as 500 mg.

A moderate kava dosage can have notable effects in alleviating generalized anxiety disorder, social anxiety, and insomnia. Generally, a dosage of 70-210 mg of kavalactone has been proven clinically effective in treating anxiety. Because the kavalactones dosage is moderate, it can reduce anxiety while leaving one alert and lucid, making it suitable for daytime use. Similar doses of between 150 and 200 mg of kavalactones, taken 30 minutes to an hour before bed, helps to encourage quicker sleep onset and better quality of sleep for people.

In general, higher doses of kavalactones promote more sociable and relaxing effects than lower doses, so in part, how much kava one should take depends on the medicinal or recreational effects sought. Personal tolerance and body chemistry affects the kava dosage needed to take for a pleasurable effect, just as different people have differing tolerances for alcohol.

The best way to find the ideal kavalactones dosage is to start with a small amount and increase the dosage over time as you become familiar with the effects it generates for you.

People who are naïve to kavalactones may not feel anything their first few times (a phenomenon called reverse tolerance), but for those who have patience in working with this herb, kava can be a marvelously gentle herb to relax with at the end of the day or turn to whenever you need a dose of calm.

> *The American Herbal Products Council has recommended that people limit their intake of kavalactones to no more than 300 milligrams per day, and not use kava for a continuous period of more than three months.*

Noble and Ignoble Kava

There are over 105 different varieties of kava grouped into two categories: Noble and Ignoble or Tudei.

The difference between Noble and Ignoble strains of kava is in the chemotype. A chemotype—also called a chemovar—is a chemically distinct entity in a plant, with differences in the composition of the secondary metabolites. Chemotypes are defined by the most abundant chemical produced by that individual plant. Different kava chemotypes are defined by the concentrations of the six major kavalactones in the kava root. Each kavalactone has an assigned number as shown in the list.

Kavalactones in Kava Root

1= desmethoxyyangonin
2= dihydrokavain
3= yangonin
4= kavain
5= dihydromethysticin
6= methysticin

A kava chemotype is "typed" based on the descending concentration of the six kavalactones within its roots. For example, cultivar such as Vanuatu Melo Melo, has a chemotype of 245361, which means it contains primarily dihydrokavain, followed in descending concentration by kavain, dihydromethysticin, yangonin, methysticin, and desmethoxyyangonin. To be classified as a "noble kava", a strain must have a chemotype that is primarily either kavain (2-4) or dihydrokavain (4-2).

The distinction between kava cultivars has to do with the effects produced in the human body by the different ratios of kavalactones. "Noble" cultivars such as Borogu, for example, are higher in smaller kavalactone molecules, such as kavain, which metabolize faster, resulting in a shorter onset and duration of physiological effects. As a result, kavain and other smaller kavalac-

Kavain is known as a "happy" kavalactone promoting mental, mood-lifting

tones have fewer side effects. Kavain is known as a "happy" kavalactone promoting mental mood-lifting effects. Kavain is known as a "happy" kavalactone promoting mental, mood-lifting effects.

In contrast, Tudei—pronounced two-day— kava, as well as wild *Piper wichmannii*, contain profuse quantities of the larger double-bonded kavalactones, like methysticin and dihydromethysticin, which take longer to metabolize and can remain active in the body for up to two days!

Some prefer Tudei kava because of its long-lasting effects, even through the increased potency is related to undesirable side effects—nausea or stomach upset, dizziness, headache, prolonged sleep, and drowsiness often lasting into the next day. Additionally, Tudei strains may contain high levels of flavokavain B, a non-kavalactone compound that may pose a hazard to the liver.

In South Pacific countries, it is understood that only noble kava strains are suitable for everyday use, whereas Tudei kavas

> *Tudei kava contain profuse quantities of the larger double-bonded kavalactones, like methysticin and dihydromethysticin, which take longer to metabolize and can remain active in the body for up to two days!*

> *Noble kava strains are suitable for everyday use, whereas Tudei kavas are reserved for ceremonial purpose and not everyday drinking.*

are reserved for ceremonial purpose and not everyday drinking. Actually, some ignoble cultivars such as Isa Kava have specific medicinal uses for conditions such as urinary tract infections and cystitis, and are also used as analgesics. Even more interesting, research has suggested that the very presence of large double-bonded kavalactones that make ignoble varieties unsuitable for casual use may be at the root of these varieties' medicinal effects, especially analgesia .

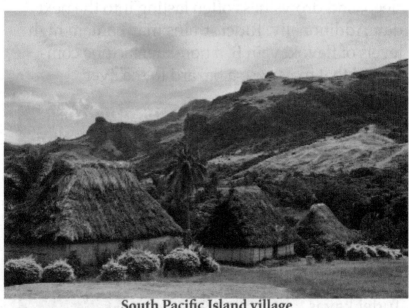

South Pacific Island village

Kava, the Plant

The leaves of Kava are few in number, simple, thin, fairly large, round or heart-shaped, pointed, smooth, green on both sides, about three to six inches in length, sometimes wider than long. The leaves tend grow in acropetal succession—a pattern of growth or movement in a downward direction from the apex of the stem to its base.

The glabrous, fleshy stems of the plant proceed from the footstalk and are usually 1 to 1-1/2 inches in diameter. They arise from the knotty crown, which is about two to six inches thick, at ground level, and in the early stages are branched. As the stem matures the lateral branches fall off, leaving conspicuous nodal scars, so that when it has reached maturity, the plant appears to consist of ten to

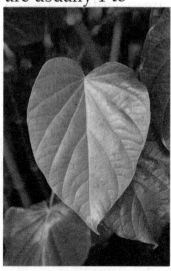

Kava leaf.

twenty separate unbranched stems arising from an extensive base or crown.

Varieties

Varieties of kava are distinguished by the height of the entire plant, the length and thickness of the joints, and the purplish or greenish tinge of stems and leaves.

* White variety: Fijian name Kasa Leka. Stem about 1 ½ to 2 inches in diameter, leaf scars broad, close together, i.e., internodes short—2-2 1/2 inches long, stem green speckled with transverse lenticels; this plant is very abundant.

* White variety: Fijian name Kasa Balavu (Yalu). Stem slender 1 1/2 inch at nodes, 3/4 inch at internodes, leaf scars small, depressed, 1/2 inch in diameter, internodes 5-10 inches long, stem pale green, lenticels linear, vertical; the plant's range is dispersed.

* White variety: Fijian name Qolobi. Stem more slender, only 1 1/4 inch at node, 3/4 to 1 inch at internode, leaf scars 1/2 to 3/4 inch, internodes 3 1/2 to 4 inches long, stem green, lenticels few, punctate, confined frequently to the upper portion of internodes. Ratio between diameter of node and internode vary marked, of the order 2:1.

- Black variety: Fijian name Kasa Leka. Stem green-black, scars 1 inch in diameter, node/internode ration 3:2, internode 3-5 inches long, lenticels dispersed, circular to transverse.

- Black variety: Fijian name Kasa Balavu. Stem slender, black, internodes 9-12 inches or more in length, 1 inch or less in diameter, scars 1/2-3/4 inch, node/internode ratio 3 :2, lenticels linear and vertical.

The white varieties are considered to be the source of the best kava, but they take longer—about four years—to attain maturity, than the black varieties, which take about 2 1/2 to 3 years. Owing however to the fact that the latter mature earlier, they have been grown on a large scale in commercial plantations.

Habitat

Kava thrives in well-drained soil and grows well as an understory crop. Too much sunlight, especially in early growth, is deleterious. Kava grows naturally where rainfall is plentiful with over 2,000 millimeters, or close to 80 inches per year.

Ideal growing conditions range from temperatures of 20 to 35 degrees Celsius, or 68 to 95 degrees Fahrenheit, with an optimum 70% to 100% relative humidity. The soil is kept loose to ensure plenty of air reaches the root, which keeps the

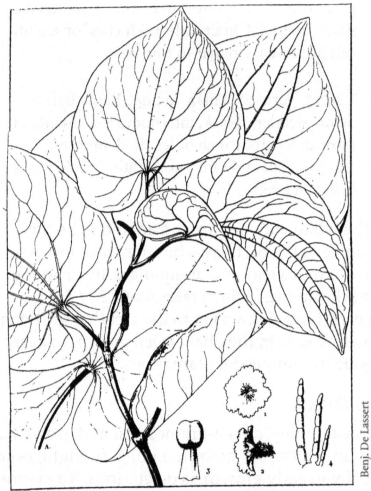

Piper Methysticum Forst.

1. *Squama floris explicata, intus visa aucta*

2. *Eadem latere visa*

3. *Stamen auctum*

4. *Pili articulait squamam vestientes, valde amplificali*

roots healthy. When the environment is too wet, the plants will develop root rot and have to be destroyed.

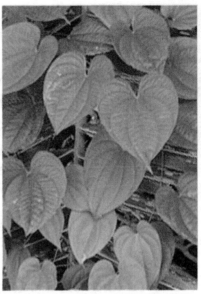

Leaves grow alternately down the length of branches in groupings of ten to thirteen from the base of the stalk.

Kava's light green, heart-shaped leaves grow alternately down the length of branches in groupings of ten to thirteen from the base of the stalk, which are approximately 30 centimeters, or about twelve inches long. The stems have green, swollen nodes that can reach up to ten inches in length. The male flowers sprout up in solitary, auxiliary, greenish white spikes up to six inches long. The flowers rise up from axils positioned opposite the leaves.

Kava's country of origin is unknown, but it is considered a native plant to many Pacific Ocean islands and grows best along the mountains of Pohnpei. The Republic of Vanuatu is informally recognized as the "home" of kava because it hosts the largest number of cultivars.

Female flowers are rare and do not produce fruit even with hand-pollination. Kava is propagated through selective breeding. There are sev-

Female flowers are rare and do not produce fruit even with hand-pollination.

eral cultivars of kava, with varying concentrations of both primary and secondary psychoactive substances. The rhizome—or rootstock—is used in modern herbal preparations, and contains the most potent of kava's psychoactive constituents.

NOTE: Only the root should be used in kava preparations for human consumption, since the tops of the plants have been shown to be toxic to the liver, while the roots have been used and proven safe over thousands of years.

Cultivation

Kava grows in shady, damp areas native to many Pacific Ocean islands.

As a tropical plant, kava kava thrives in conditions with lots of water, sun and moderate humidity and temperatures of 68-80 degrees Fahrenheit—20-25 Celsius. Because it usually grows under the jungle canopy, kava does best with partial shade rather than full sun, especially when young. It grows densely to a height of about 20 feet. It develops slowly and does not bear flowers—which consist of catkins—for the first time only after 2 1/2 to 3 years. The flowers, which are rarely found, are dioecious.

Monoecious plants have both male and female reproductive parts on the same flower, while dioecious plants produce male and female parts on different flowers. This means that while a monoecious plant may pollinate itself, dioecious plants require a partner to achieve pollination.

Domesticated kava—Piper methysticum—plants are sterile because they do not produce seeds. New plants are grown from cuttings or the root bundle of the plant. Kava plants propagate easily by cuttings and takes two years to produce the treasured roots.

It is fairly easy to propagate kava plants by dividing a healthy kava plant's root bundle. The kava plant is carefully removed from the garden bed and excess soil is brushed off. The root mass is divided where smaller root masses branch off. The offshoots are removed and the

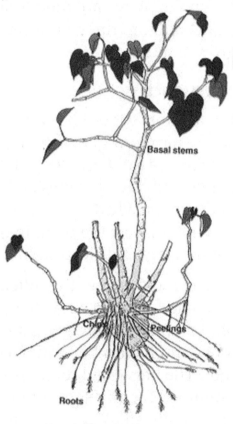

Kava roots.

plant is repotted in loose soil in smaller containers. Moisture, which is essential, is maintained to get the cuttings to successfully root. Coconut husks, a common hydroponic growing medium, help to regulate water. Husks are mixed into loose rich soil and about ten percent garden-grade sand is added.

Even though kava is happiest in super-sunny, tropical regions of the world, it is best grown in partial shade. Adequate shade is especially important with young kava cuttings because the sun can easily burn and dry out the leaves. When the plants are three years old, they can be moved into full sun to encourage maximum growth rates.

Harvesting

Kava plants should be two to three years old before harvesting. Harvesting before at least one year of age can harm, even kill the plant. Older plants will have accumulated more kavalactones in the roots, which are the active phytochemicals that protect the plant in the wild and give it anti-anxiety and sleep-inducing qualities.

The roots are gently pulled from the soil, dirt is washed off, and a few lateral roots are snipped off. Lateral roots are generally higher in kavalactones and have a better flavor than the vertical root. The harvested roots should be carefully examined for any signs of mold. The fresh roots are cut into small sections, and dried.

Kava Chemistry

The earliest chemical examination of kava root was made by M. Cuzent in 1860. About the same time Gobley, in collaboration with O'Rorke, found the air-dried rootstock to contain: 26 percent cellulose, 49 percent starch, one percent-mcthysticin—a crystalline principle—one percent, two percent acrid balsamic resin combined with an essential oil of a citron-yellow color, fifteen percent moisture, and seven percent of gum and substances of minor importancewhich include four percent ash or mineral matter of which one percent is potassium chloride and three percent iscalcium carbonate, and traces of magnesium, silicon, argillaceous earth and iron oxide. Tannin has never been found.

According to Gobley, the active principle resides in the balsamic resin, contents of which have been variously estimated as between three and eight percent, although the figure depends on the age of the rootstock, and probably also on the methods used for its determination.

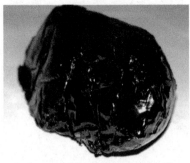

A drop of kava resin on the tongue produces numbness and a soapy taste.

According to investigations made by L. Lewin around 1866, a drop of kawaic resin on the tongue produces numbness, and a fatty or soapy taste. He concluded that kawaic resin is the only constituent of the rootstock that has an anaesthetic effect.

Lewin isolated what he termed alpha-kawaic resin and beta-kawaic resin, the former being the more potent. He found that this substance caused anaesthesia of the mucous membranes in a similar way to cocaine, and that if a tiny piece, even as small as a needle-head, of a mixture of both resins were put into the eye of an animal, a complete anaesthesia of the cornea and conjunctiva is produced within three minutes or even sooner. However Lewin did not succeed in isolating the principle in a crystalline condition.

A painstaking systematic investigation of the herb was made by W. Borscht and his co-workers during the years 1913 to 1933. Although they isolated a number of chemical substances from the rootstock and their structure determined, they did not succeed in identifying the main active principle.

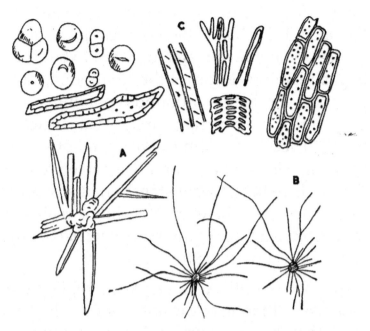

Microcystals Formed in Kava Root

A. Crystals of methysticin obtained by treatment on secitons of the rootstock or its powder with alcohol, the cyystals being of a light yellow colour, attaining a length of 0.16 mm. and becoming violet red through the addition of sulphuric acid. **B.** Crystals of ethysticic acid obtained upon heating a small quantity of the powder with one or two drops of solution of potassium hydroxide and adding with dilute alcohol and allowing the slide to stand for 24 hours. Crystals of methysticin can also be obtained by sublimination, providing the powder has been acted on previously with dilute sulphuric acid, emulsim or saliva—*After Tunmann, in Gehe & Co's, Handelsbericht, 1912; From Henry Kraemer's Scientific and Applied Pharmacognosy, 1920, pp. 153-154.*

Among the substances isolated were methysticin $C_{15}H_{14}O_5$, yangonin $C_{15}H_{14}O_3$ and kawain $C_{14}H_{14}O_3$, which is a resinous substance, insoluble in water, but said to be soluble in gastric juices. Many of the compounds are lactones—organic compounds containing oxygen—and have a certain similarity in structure. Bosche tried to confirm the structure of kawain by synthesis, but failed and was forced to admit that none of his new substances had any physiological activity whatever. Nor did he realize that dihydrokawain plays an important part in the typical effect of the entire herb.

It was not until A. G. van Veen applied the modern technique of the adsorption column in 1938, that the active principle was finally and rather easily obtained, namely in crystalline condition by a combination of an appropriate method of extraction with adsorption analysis—chromatography.

The most suitable adsorbent appeared to be well dried "acid clay", a particular argillaceous earth produced in Java; other sorts of alumina, franconite were not suitable. The ultimate purification with petrol-ether/ether mixtures as developer was much more troublesome. This crystallizable principle has been termed marindinin $C_{14}H_{16}O_3$, melting point 60° C, named after the tribe of the Marindinese of Netherlands New-Guinea.

It was subsequently shown to be identical with dihydrokawain, previously isolated by Borsche from the kawa resin, and is a tasteless, unsaturated lactone. It is soluble in alcohol and ether. This substance is narcotic only if it is brought into the form of a fine emulsion.

Van Veen made several tests as to the soporific effect of marindinin on pigeons and small monkeys. Monkeys have the unpleasant habit of continuing to resist as long as possible the effect of a kava dose, which necessitates a very high dose. Van Veen arrived at the conclusion that the only physiologically active constituent of the rootstock was dihydrokawain—marindinin, but likewise did not succeed in synthesizing the substance.

Other investigators also examined kava and found that it contained no glycosides, nor were alkaloids detected in the resin, although nitrogen was present. Prof. Dr. Rudolf Hansel of Berlin undertook to test kava rootstock as to soporific properties. He applied

The formulae of dihydromethysticin and dihydro-methysticic acid.

a chromatographic method for the isolation of die ingredients, and he identified another sedative principle of the herb, dihydromethysticin. Doses of 50 to 200 mg/kg dihydrokawain and dihydromethysticin induced sleep in white mice and rats 20 minutes after application through a stomach tube.

Hansel found that dihydrokawain—which is insoluble in water—is about 95 per cent soluble in groundnut oil at a temperature of 37° C. Hansel therefore, dissolved this ingredient in hot groundnut oil, cooled it to about 30° C. and ap-

dihydromethysticin   dihydromethysticic acid

plied the oily solution. But as to dihydromethysticin, no such solution could be obtained by this method, and Hansel had to emulsify the rubbed crystals with gum arabic and groundnut oil in water.

Hansel arrived at the same conclusion as Van Veen did previously, namely that dihydrokawain—marindinin—constitutes the central principle of kava rootstock. Hansel identified dihydromethysticin as another sedative ingredient of the rootstock of kava. Dihydromethysticin does not act as quickly as dihydrokawain,

however the effect
of the former lasts
longer. The other
ingredients were
found to be inac-
tive. From 1 kg
finely milled kava
rootstock, Hansel

Carbon-skeleton of the typical
kava constituents.

obtained 3.3 grams dihydrokawain and 4 grams
dihydromethysticin.

The chemical formula of the kava ingredients—the 5 pyronone derivatives—is not com-
plicated: a benzene ring is linked through a
two-carbon side-chain with a pyronone ring;
four of these ingredients—the kava lactones—
namely methysticin, kawain, dihydrokawain
and dihydromethysticin belong to the y-pyro-
none group, yangonin belongs to the y-pyro-
none group.

The unsaturated lactone ring is principally
responsible for the narcotic effect of the kava
ingredients. We know from other unsaturated 6-membcred lactones—as e.g. in the case
of coumarin, and in the oil present in massoy
bark, that unsaturated lactones can have such
an effect, though in coumarin the effect is much
weaker.

For this reason it is remarkable, that in the
case of the active principles of the kava herb—
i.e., the dihydro-derivatives, viz. dihydrokawain

and dihydromcthysticin—contrary to other lactones—the twofold binding in the carbon chain
between the benzene ring on the one side and
the 6-membered lactone ring on the other aide
is hydrated; after application of methysticin and
kawnm-compounds with intact lactone ring, no
soporific effect could be observed!

Synthesis

In 1942, K. Zieglar discovered a method to bro-
minate a system containing double bonds, without attacking these double bonds. By Hansel's
systematic investigation he arrived at the conclusion, that bromosuccinimide is an ideal bro-
minating agent. This reaction was the origin of a
simple synthesis of kawain.

F. Kngl and 0. A. de Bruin were the first to
use this synthesis, and applied the method to the
synthesis of auxin-b analogs. The synthesis was
successful and, it was thought, kawain had been
synthesized for the first time. However, another
synthesis along a different route had been an-
nounced by E. R. H. Jams, and the melting points of
the substances, obtained from both methods, were
found to be identical. Therefore, there are two ways
to synthesize kawain. Dihydrokawain was also
synthesized, which had the melting point 76° C.

*The unsaturated lactone ring
is principally responsible
for the narcotic effect of the
kava ingredients.*

Conclusions

Though the problem of the synthesis of kawain and methysticin is solved, this does not provide products with the same physiological activity. This is probably because the action of kava is due not to one substance, but to a mixture of substances acting synergistically, *It should be realized that one substance is so dependent on the presence of another, that the plant or the part of the plant used in its entirety, often yields much better re-mits in therapy than any of its isolated substances.* some of which are of secondary importance, but still of real value, and including infinitesimal quantities of the inorganic ingredients, usually occurring as salts in plants, and which are termed trace minerals.

It is a fact, that most medicinal plants owe their therapeutic activity largely—but not always exclusively!—to the presence of an active principle or principles. But it should be realized that one substance is so dependent on the presence of another, that the plant or the part of the plant used in its entirety, often yields much better remits in therapy than any of its isolated substances. Indeed, the so-called "physiologically inert" material in plants often constitutes an indispensable factor, and this "inert" material is by no means needless bulk. This situation seems to be particularly true in the case of kava rootstock, because investigation has rendered it probable, that the potassium chloride—a salt present to the extent of about 0.04 per cent, as found by Gobley—stands in a peculiar relation to the resin molecule, being apparently in chemical combination with it.

We have seen that most herbs contain more than one active principle, and that the principles present are similar in structure,and are mostly an extremely complex mixture of substances of quite different character. We learned from Hansel's investigations, that as regards kava rootstock dihydrokawain is the most potent, but not the sole active principle.

Although the active principles of kava rootstock are narcotics, for them to be active it is essential that they be brought into the form of a fine emulsion, before they can exert their narcotic properties.

As in the case of quite a number of herbs, the chemical processes employed in the isolation of medicinal organic substances can produce disturbances in the metabolism and structure of kava rootstock and, therefore, in its properties, which are retained when the herb is used in its crude state, in the form of a suitable galenical preparation. In this connection it should be realized that, when a medicine is prepared through infusion or decoction of a dried plant or a part of a plant, the enzymes—complex protein materials which act in the living cells of plants as a catalyst, and increase metabolic activity and breakdown of the substrate—can be destroyed. But when extracts or tinctures are prepared by cold maceration, the enzymes are preserved. In fact, in some instances the value of a herb is due entirely to the products of enzyme action. In this connection it should be pointed out here, that on the South Pacific islands, kava beverages are always prepared with cold water or coconut milk.

Although the active principles of kava rootstock are narcotics, for them to be active it is essential that they be brought into the form of a fine emulsion, before they can exert their narcotic properties. This is the main explanation of the differential action of the herb, when used as a drink prepared after grating or pounding and macerating in water, and a beverage prepared by chewing

It is possible and highly advantageous to replace saliva by water, without loss of narcotic activity, but the finely milled material should be rubbed for a sufficiently long time in a mortar or with the aid of modern techniques; it should then be emulsified with a little oil—not a heavy oil, but a light oil like olive oil or coconut oil—and lecithin, so that a milky substance is obtained.

The general structure of the kavalactones, without the R1-R2 -O-CH2-O- bridge and with all possible C=C double bonds shown.

A total of 18 different kavalactones—or kava-pyrones—have been identified to date, at least 15 of which are active. However, six of them, including kavain, dihydrokavain, methysticin, dihydromethysticin, yangonin, and desmethoxyyangonin, have been determined to be responsible for about 96 percent of the plant's pharmacological activity. Some minor constituents, including three chalcones, flavokavain A, flavokavain B, and flavokavain C, have also been identified, as well as a toxic alkaloid pipermethystine, which is not present in the consumable parts of the plant.

Pharmacodynamics

The following pharmacological actions have been reported for kava and/or its major active constituents:

- Potentiation of GABAA receptor activity.

- Inhibition of the reuptake of norepinephrine and possibly also of dopamine.

- Binding to the CB1 receptor.

- Inhibition of voltage-gated sodium channels and voltage-gated calcium channels.

- Monoamine oxidase B reversible inhibition.

Receptor binding assays with botanical extracts have revealed direct interactions of leaf extracts of kava (which appear to be more active than root extracts) with the GABA—i.e., main—binding site of the GABAA receptor, the D2 receptor, the μ-opioid receptors, and the H1 and H2 receptors. Weak interaction with the 5-HT6 and 5-HT7 receptors and the benzodiazepine site of the GABAA receptor was also observed.

Potentiation of GABAA receptor activity may underlie the anxiolytic effects of kava, while elevation of dopamine levels in the nucleus accumbens likely underlie the moderately psychotropic effects the plant can produce.

Changes in the activity of 5-HT neurons could explain the sleep-inducing action. However, failure of the GABAA receptor inhibitor flumazenil to reverse the anxiolytic effects of kava in mice suggests that benzodiazepine-like effects are not contributing to the pharmacological profile of kava extracts.

Caution: Heavy, long-term use of kava has been found to not reduce ability in cognitive tests, but has been associated with elevated liver enzymes.

Kava Root

The rhizome or rootstock, scraped clean at place of origin from its outer corky layer, is found in commerce in pieces usually weighing from two to ten lbs. The root is cut and dried into segments varying from one to two inches in length and one to two inches in diameter. The rhizome is longitudinally wrinkled and has large circular root scars; externally yellowish-gray, internally whitish with light-brown or dark-brown spots; fracture of small pieces short and somewhat splintery; fracture of thicker pieces tough; central portions porous with a large pith and a distinctly radiate xylem; irregularly twisted wood bundles separated by broad medullary

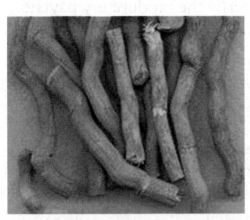

The root is cut and dried into segments varying from one to two inches in length and one to two inches in diameter.

rays of a sclerenchymatous nature, so that under the thin bark—underlaid by a very thin cortical layer—the wood bundles form distinct meshes.

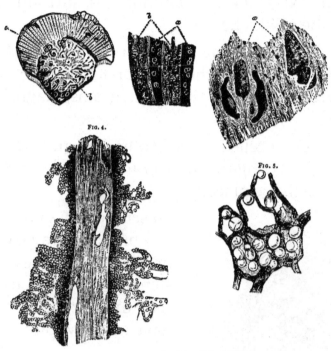

From a drawing by Mr. Alfred White

Drawing by Mr. Alfred While

Fig 1. Cross section of the item (natural size), which it composed of an outer layer (a), in which plates of woody and vascular tissue alternate with masses of small cells, filled with starch grains, and likewise a few vessels; and of a central accumulation of cells, filled with starch grains; through these pass large bundles of vascular and woody tissue.

Fig. 2. Represents the outer layer, magnified 12x; (a) being the woody and vascular plates, and (b) those of cellular tissue.

Fig. 3. Is a portion of the cellular mass, magnified 12x; (a) the vascular bundles, surrounded by the cellula tissue.

Fig. 4. A longitudinal section of one of the vascular bundles (of the central part), with its surrounding cells and starch grains; magnified 25x.

Fig. 5. A few cells - of the center -, magnified 200x; showing the manner in which the grains of starch are placed.

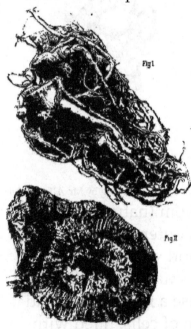

Fig1

FigⅡ

KAVA RHIZOME
From Lewm, L. - Piper melhysti-
cum, Berlin **1886.** *Paul Geissler*
Kunstwerkstatt, Berlin

Unscraped rhizome is of a blackish-gray color externally. Pieces of stem are more woody than the rhizome and have a hollow pith.

The roots, when not removed, are often twelve inches or more long—sometimes up to six feet, more or less fibrous and of a grayish-brown color.

Older rhizomes can be distinguished by numerous splits and holes, caused by the destruction of the parenchyma tissues.

A drop of sulphuric acid, applied to the surface of the rhizome, produc-es a deep cher-ry-red color. The rhizome and the

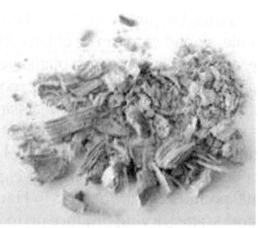

Kava Rootstock.

stem abound in wood fibres, which—with starch constitute its great bulk. From the edges of the pithy center, consisting of cells filled with starch grains, proceed plates of woody and vascular tissue, alter-nating with small cells filled with starch.

Harvesting the Rootstock

Rootstocks can be dug up from time to time as required. For ceremonies, the natives preferred the fresh rootstock to the dried, though it has been found that the latter is nearly as strong. Sometimes the stems are also harvested.

The rootstock—just below the surface of the ground, and for two feet or so becomes three to five inches thick at maturity, which is about 2 1/2 to 4 years after planting. In a patch of kava, the roots eventually become a heavy, knotted mass, and such a patch is highly prized, for the rootstock gathers strength and flavor with age.

When the plant is cultivated on a commercial scale, a good crop can be obtained in three or four years after planting, each plant averaging three pounds of dried rootstock. The rootstock is full-grown after a period of six years and then its weight sometimes exceeds 20 pounds, but it seldom is left untouched until such a long time has elapsed. Roots about 20 years old can have a weight of more, than 100 pounds, but arc a rarity. In Hawaii, many rootstocks, after drying produce up to 20 pounds. in three or four years after planting.

The older rootstocks and stems carry a higher percentage of the active principles than the younger parts.

To prepare them for the market, the rootstocks and the underground basal parts are scraped, in order to remove the outer coat. Then they are cut into pieces and dried in the sun, or in an airy spot on a platform over a fireplace. In Hawaii, drying is done in a nearly airtight shed, heated by Ohia logs, after the rootstock is first chopped into small pieces, each weighing 1/2 to 1-1/2 ounce or shredded. Diseased portions are usually cut out. During the drying process the weight diminishes to between one fourth and one sixth.

> *The older rootstocks and stems carry a higher percentage of the active principles than the younger parts.*

Effects of Kava Drinking

The effect of the beverage prepared by chewing is different from the beverage prepared by macerating after grating or pounding the rootstock. Chewing produces the strongest effect because it produces the finest particles. Fresh, undried kava produces a stronger beverage than dry kava. The strength also depends on the species and techniques of cultivation.

The kava brew prepared by grating or pounding and macerating in cold water is a comparatively harmless *tonic and stimulant.* The kava brew prepared by grating or pounding beverage is often given to the sick and convalescent.

When the brew is prepared by chewing—mixed with saliva. the effect is *narcotic* Taken *in moderation,* kava prepared by chewing has a peculiar, narcotic action. It paralyzes the sensory nerves

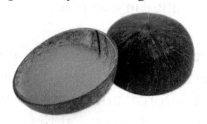

Brew in traditional coconut cup.

Effects of Kava

I felt the first effects of kava in about five minutes. The muscles throughout my body became softer, more elastic. My face became relaxed and pliable as subtle tension seemed to drain out of my facial muscles. I became aware of my breathing, which felt deeper, slightly more full, and definitely more pleasurable than usual. Over the course of the next few minutes a sensuous wave of relaxation washed slowly over my entire body like India ink spreading over while paper. My visual and auditory acuity also became heightened. I noticed subtle gradations of light spreading out from the dinner candles to brilliant blue, yellow-white at the base of the flame, growing soft and diffuse in gray tones as it reached the farthest corners of the dining room. I observed variations in the color and depth of shadows along the floor and ceiling. Outside sounds became pronounced. The chirping of crickets was sharp and high. I was acutely aware of the rich and varied tones of the voices of my friends. The barely audible touch of finger tips grasping drinking glasses and the occasional gentle shuffle of shoes on the polished hardwood floor as my friends shifted the positions of their legs. My mind was lucid and clear. The overall effects was one of great pleasure and complete mental alertness. It was delightful.

Chris Kilhan
*Kava: Medicine
Hunting in Paradise*

and first stimulates, then paralyzes the muscles, particularly affecting the lower limbs. It increases the force, but decreases the rapidity of the heart's action and at first stimulates, then depresses the respiratory center.

A moderately potent kava drink causes effects within 10–20 minutes that last for about two and a half hours, but can be felt for up to eight hours. Some report longer-term effects up to two days after ingestion, including a feeling of mental clarity, patience, and an ease of acceptance. The effects of kava are most often compared to alcohol, or benzodiazepines.

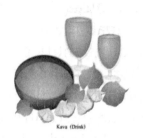

Kava (Drink)

The sensations, in order of appearance, are slight tongue and lip numbing, mildly talkative and sociable behavior, clear thinking, calmness, relaxed muscles, and a sense of well-being. The numbing of the mouth is caused by the two kavalactones kavain and dihydrokavain, which cause the contraction of the blood vessels in these areas, acting as a local topical anesthetic.

The effects of a kava drink vary widely with the particular chemotype of kava plant and amount. A potent drink results in a faster on-set with a lack of stimulation; the user's eyes become more sensitive, and the person soon becomes somnolent. Sleep is often restful and pronounced periods of sleepiness correlate to the amount and potency of kava consumed. Many people reportedly experience deep sleep and rather vivid dreams after drinking moderate amounts of kava.

In contrast to alcohol, the kava brew does not impair mental alertness, until sleep comes. A small quantity gives rise to a euphoric state of short duration. People drinking kava brew do not talk loudly, fight or become quarrelsome; on the contrary, they are generally tranquil and friendly. In fact, the drinker manifests an unwillingness to be annoyed.

But when a people drinks *too much* of kava brew, their vision becomes disturbed, as the pupils are enlarged and react very slowly to light. They stagger because walking is difficult or impossible. They just want to sleep. Kava has been described as "the most powerful soporific in existence"!

The universal opinion that kava possesses intoxicating powers, is not correct. Kava is a spinal rather than a cerebral depressant, since the higher nerve centers retain their normal functional activity. It steadies the pulse and does not raise the temperature. It also possesses diaphoretic, and slightly diuretic and stomachic properties.

Small quantities bring on a state of happy carelessness, content, and well-being appears without any physical or mental excitation.

The qualities of the beverage are not lasting, although the drug contains sleep-producing

active princi-
ples and pro-
duces muscu-
lar weakness.
A wine glass
full of strong
kava beverage
is sufficient
to produce
a profound

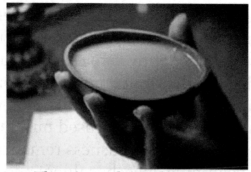

**There is much ritual with the
drinking of the brew.**

dreamless sleep in about a half hour. in a soporific drug this quality is a very good one. After
a few hours, by next morning, the kava drinker
awakens feeling rested and fit. Strength is re-
stored.

The kava brew is neither an alcoholic beverage nor a psychedelic drug. Nevertheless, it
does have sedative and anesthetic properties.
The effects of the kava brew vary from person
to person. Generally when taken in a small
amount, the drinker experiences a mild feeling of sleepiness and drowsiness, relaxation of
the body and the muscles, feelings of happiness, and numbness of the mouth, tongue and
throat. When taken in a larger quantity, the
kava brew may cause the loss of muscle control, sleepiness, the reddening of the eyes and
the dilation of the pupils, and a general feeling
of sickness.

A carefully prepared kava beverage taken in small quantity and not too strong produces a state of happy carelessness, content, and well-being without any physical or mental excitation. It is a real euphoric state, which is accompanied by an increased muscular efficiency. Reason and consciousness remain unaffected. At the beginning speech is fluent and lively and the hearing becomes more sensible to subtle impressions. Kava has a soothing effect. Those who drink it are never choleric, angry, aggressive or noisy, as in the case of alcohol.

In this form kava brew is a stimulating beverage after imbibing, where hardships can be endured more easily. It refreshes the fatigued body and brightens and sharpens the intellectual faculties. Appetite is augmented, especially if it is taken half an hour before meals.

If enough of the active principle is ingested peculiar narcotic phenomena appear. In the first report of Cook's travels it is stated that some of the crew had drunk of the beverage, and that effects were observed similar to those of a large dose of a spirituous liquor or of opium.

After the consumption of greater quantities, however, the limbs become weary, the muscles seem to be out of control of the will, the gait is slow and unsteady, and the subject appears half drunk. An urgent desire to lie down manifests itself. The eye sees objects before it but is unable to identify them with precision. In the same way the ears hear everything, but the individual may not be able to account for what is heard. Everything becomes more and more diffuse. The drinker succumbs to fatigue, and experiences a strong desire to sleep, becoming somnolent and finally falling asleep.

The sleep is similar to that produced by alcohol, out of which the individual can be awakened only with difficulty. If moderate quantities have been consumed it occurs twenty to thirty minutes later, and lasts from two to eight hours according to the degree of habituation of the subject. If the beverage is concentrated, containing a large amount of the resinous components of kava, intoxication comes on much more rapidly. Occasionally a short state of nervous trembling occurs before they fall asleep. No excitation precedes these symptoms. Unlike with alcohol, there is no after-effect or hang-over.

The Kava Brew

Kava brew is a habit-forming drink, and said to be irresistible once its taste is acquired. Today kava brew is macerated and softened in cold water after having been grated or pounded. It is relatively innocuous, comparable to beer drinking, an effect referred to as a tonic and stimulant, whereas that of the beverage prepared by chewing is definitely narcotic.

There are two methods of preparing the beverage: By chewing and thorough pounding or grating the rootstock, and macerating in cold water or coconut milk. Traditionally Pacific islanders prepared

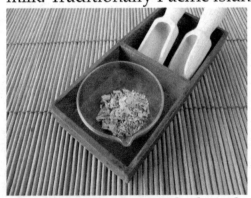

the kava brew in a manner that today would be considered disgusting and unsanitary. The cleaned and scraped rootstocks, called "waka", the roots,

Ceremonial kava tray with cleaned chipped root.

and the extreme base of the stem, called "lewe-na", were beaten on a stone until reduced to fragments.

Chewers

Pretty young girls with rosy lips and pearly teeth were chose for their prepossessing appearance, and young lads who occupied a certain social rank towards the man, for whom they performed the office. The girls, sitting cross-legged on mats on the ground, breast bare, with flowers coquettishly stuck in their hair, and only a very slight drapery of native cloth—often a band curiously worked of grass and bark of different colors—round the waist, made a very pretty picture; the girls' beauty was supposed to counteract the filthy method of preparing the "nectar".

The chewers spat the kava into a bowl, where it was mixed with coconut milk. It was believed that the chewing procedure blended the root with enzymes in the saliva that promoted the extraction of the active ingredients of the root and generally produced a much tastier brew. In most of the Pacific Islands this method of letting

The root fragments were chewed by women, preferably virgins, with strong jaws and good teeth.

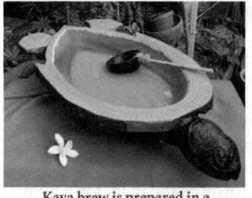

Kava brew is prepared in a traditonal native bowl.

girls and boys or other chew the rootstock is now forbidden by law, owing to its liability to spread disease. It also destroys the teeth in the course of time.

Saliva

When masticated, the mash was sialagogue—promoted secretion of saliva—and caused a burning sensation and numbing of the tongue. The saliva tended to be more viscid than usual. After diligently reducing to a soft, comminuted mass with saliva, the quid was spit into a half-coconut shell or calabash—a bottled gourd—and, together with other chewed quids, placed in a bowl. The bowl was a circular, shallow wooden vessel standing upon many short legs. Bowls vary in size from nine to 36 inches in diameter.

The mass was then mixed with cold water or coconut milk until it reached the right consistency. The supernatant liquid formed the kava potion, froth resembling soap suds. Typically the mass was stirred by hand and then cleared by stirring with a bundle of the very narrow strips of the fibers, obtained from the inner bark of a *Hibiscus tiliaceus* tree. This dexterous manipulation was considered an art, often performed very gracefully.

Working the Concoction

The concoction was then strained through coconut fiber, squeezing the pieces of masticated root until all the juices were blended with the water. This liquid was then decanted into another bowl for consumption. Traditionally the beverage prepared by chewing was reserved for religious rates and only drunk by the grown-up males. The beverage is astringent and peculiarly pungent, but not bitter. Women and children were excluded from the drinking parties.

The liquid was then wrung out by kneading the fibers three or four times through dry grass or through coconut husks so that the woody disintegrated pulp and dregs were caught in the strainer. Finally the strainer was again dipped into the contents of the bowl and squeezed out as a sponge to fill the cups.

The beverage prepared by chewing is refreshing, with cleansing properties. This drink is served with a special ceremony. Kava is an integral part of the religious and social life of the natives; drinking it is essential on occasions of hospitality and feasting, but the ritual varies considerably in the various islands or groups of islands. The drinking of kava is more a kind of ceremonial rite than debauchery.

Tanoa Bowls

Traditional kava ceremonies used beautifully carved and polished bowls, called *tanoa*, often cut out of a solid section of the dark-brown wood of the *Vesi*, the Fijian name for *Afzelia bijuga*.

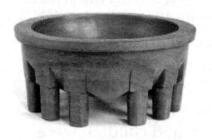

Tanoa Bowl

The bowls can hold from 4 to 10 pints. In very old and much used bowls, a grayish-white or yellowish-green crust with a bluish or purplish glitter was formed in the course of time, which finally resulted in a pearly-bluish color. After a period of 20 years, this coating was sometimes half an inch thick, and looked as if the bowl had been inlaid with mother-of-pearl.

The mother-of-pearl look is formed by the resinous substance kawain, which is insoluble in water, and is set free in the chewed mass. As the chewed mass is mixed with water and stirred, particles of the yellowish or greenish-yellow kawain, together with particles of the grayish powder of the rootstock, stick to the kawain, together with particles of the grayish powder of the rootstock, stick to the inside of the bowl, and so this coating is gradually formed. A similar coating is formed in coconut shells used as drinking cups, which are scraped and rubbed with stones under water into a thin, highly polished cup. Neither the bowls nor the cups are ever wiped dry after having contained kava, but are simply emptied.

Modern Method of Preparation

Nowadays kava beverage is prepared in a more hygienic way, by grating or pounding the rootstock between two stones—with a small boulder on the concave top of a larger boulder—or by pulverizing in a blender. It is mixed with cold water, and thoroughly stirred for at least five minutes. Generally about half an ounce of the powdered rootstock is mixed into one pint of water or coconut milk. Strength of the liquid is liable to considerable variation.

Extraction of the psychoactive compounds from the kava root is performed by leaching the root into liquid such as water or milk. Both work well for kava extractions, since the kavalactones leach into either fluid. However, the best liquid to draw out the active constituents of kava should contain a healthy amount of fat, such as cow's milk, goat's milk, soy milk or coconut milk. Simply put, using a fluid containing fat is the best way to prepare kava extractions, in addition to making a delicious kava drink.

Kava is now readily available in specialty shops and online as a whole root and powder. Kavalactones are insoluble in water and are destroyed by heat. The rootstock should be powdered and then infused in *cold* water for a few minutes. Then it is carefully squeezed through a cloth to release the activity constituents from the root stock fiber.

Never use hot liquid when preparing the kava brew, because the high temperature destroys kava's main active ingredients known as kavalactones—the psychoactive components of kava that provide the drink with its relaxing properties.

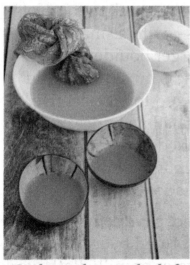

In the modern method of making the brew the root is grond up and squeezed through water.

The flavor and strange numbing sensation of Kava is a disincentive for regular usage. There are many quality Kava tablets available for those times when the full Kava experience is neither desired nor needed.

This modern way of preparing the kava brew produces a drink that is less potent and different in action from that obtained through the traditional practice of chewing. Chewing is necessary to reduce the rootstock to minute particles if a *narcotic* effect is to be obtained.

Because the active principles are insoluble in water, but liberated in a process of emulsification, the beverage prepared by merely macerating the rootstock in water has an effect quite different from the beverage prepared by chewing. This distinction is important.

Whichever way the beverage is prepared, the brew becomes stale within a few hours, so it should be consumed as soon as possible at one sitting in accordance with traditional custom.

Usually a little water or coconut milk is drunk after the kava to rinse the mouth and a morsel of food eaten. Eating too much food tends to produce nausea. Kava grated or pounded and prepared by macerating in water, is often drunk copiously and requires less caution.

Preparing Brew at Home

Kava brew is easy and fun to prepare with friends, especially when following the traditional squeezing process. Make sure to use only the root, which contains the highest concentration of kavalactones when preparing the kava brew. The small lateral roots that grow along the surface of the soil are especially loaded with kavalactones.

The potency of kava brew is determined by three factors—species, age of root, and method of preparation. The variety of species is of primary significance. Age of the root makes a difference in the potency. Roots are not mature or ready for drinking until at least five years old. As the root gets older the concentration of kavalactones increases as the root increases in size.

Preparation

The rootstock should be powdered and then infused in cold water for a few minutes. Then it is vigorously squeezed through a cloth to release the active constituents from the root stock fiber.

Avoid Heat

When making kava brew, it's important to use water that is less than 140 degrees Farhrenheit because the root's active kavalactones break down at higher temperatures.

How To Prepare Kava Brew

1. For one part kava, use two parts water and one part coconut milk.

2. Pour lukewarm to the touch—not hot—water into a large bowl.

3. Put the dry kava in a strainer bag and immerse the bag in water.

4. Knead and squeeze the kava into the bowl of liquid while applying a lot of pressure for 10-15 minutes.

Use one to two ounces—two to four tablespoons—of powder per person. Put the powdered root into the strainer bag, hold its edges together at the top to prevent the powder from escaping, and immerse the bag with root into a bowl of cool water. As a rule of thumb use two ounces of powder to a quart of water. Knead the kava under the water and squeeze, then immerse it again in

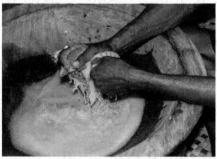

Squeezing water through the root in the bag.

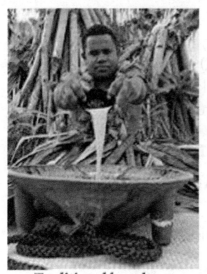

Traditional kava brew preparation.

the water. The kneading is the most critical step in the entire process!

The kava will feel oily at first due to kava-lactone levels. Repeat the kneading process until the kava no longer feels oily. The water will have the appearance of mud.

Add Oil

The kava brew is a suspension of root matter in cool water. However, kavalactones are fat-soluble rather than water-soluble. So the liquid needs to contain fat to dissolve the kavalactones, which is accomplished by adding a fatty liquid such as milk or coconut milk to the mix.

Extraction of the psychoactive compounds from the kava root is performed by leaching the root into liquid such as water or milk. The squeezing produces an emulsion where small droplets of the lipid-like compounds are suspended in water. Then when fat is added—such as in cow's milk, goat's milk, soy milk or coconut milk—the psychoactive compounds, which are fat-soluble, are absorbed into the fat. Simply put, using a fluid containing fat is the best way to prepare kava extractions, in addition to making a delicious kava drink.

Quickie Brew

Many enthusiasts replace the kneading by using an electric blender. For a "kava quickie" put three tablespoons kava root powder in a blender with three cups of water. Add a teaspoon of vegetable oil, which makes for a smoother tasting drink and helps to emulsify the kavalactones in the water.

Blend on "High" for two to three minutes. Strain the brew through a cheesecloth strainer bag, a sock, or scrap of a T-shirt or through a fine tea strainer for a more pleasant smoother tasting drink. You may want to use more or less water according to your taste. Keep leftovers in the refrigerator.

This makes a great iced drink. In fact, one of the best ways to make kava taste better is to drink it cold after putting the prepared drink in the refrigerator for a few hours. Leaving it in the fridge overnight seems to mellow the taste even more.

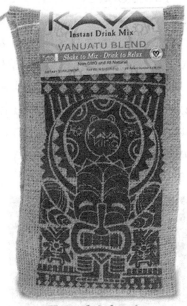

Drink slowly to allow the lactones to be absorbed directly into

Kava drink mix.

mucus membranes of your mouth for immediate effects that cause the pleasant tingling sensation that kava is famous for.

Some people add a few slices of fresh ginger root to the blender for a spicy taste. Sweetening the brew with a bit of honey is good, as is using maple syrup.

Taste

The taste of kava brew is pungent, but not bitter; even the confirmed kava drinker makes a face and shakes his head when he swallows a potion.The odor of kava is faint but lilac-like and usually pleasurable. The color is grey to tan to opaque yellow-greenish.

Traditionally, each serving of this prepared kava was swallowed in one or two quick gulps from a coconut shell and always with thoughts of giving thanks. It is a good idea to space servings at least 10 minutes apart as the kavain, the kavalactone highest in most Hawaiian kava varieties is usually felt quite soon after drinking, but other kavalactones effects may not register for 20 minutes or so.

Generally, people drink Kava Kava brews __instead of__ alcohol, rather than with it.

A strong kava drink is normally followed by a hot meal. The meal traditionally follows some time after the drink to allow time for the psychoactives to be absorbed into the bloodstream.

Kava or Alcohol

It was generally assumed that the secret of the action of kava lay in its mode of preparation. It was said that during mastication the saliva transformed the starch of the root into sugar, and that this by fermentation turned into alcohol. The kavalactones are also soluble in alcohol but mixing kava with alcohol can be precarious because each propincipates the other, rendering the effects of each stronger. Drinking kava with alcohol may also increase alcoholic effects. With this being said, common side effects of alcohol such as vomiting and drowsiness may occur more readily if consumed together with kava. It is advisable to consult a doctor if you are taking any other medications, alcohol, or drugs with kava

This brings us to a discussion of what actually happens to the liver when kava and

> ### Active Substances & Their Actions
>
> *It was generally assumed that the secret of the action of kava lay in its mode of preparation. It was said that during mastication the saliva transformed the starch of the root into sugar, and that this by fermentation turned into alcohol.*

alcohol are used in combination. The liver makes use of the enzyme CYP 2E1 for the metabolizing of alcohol. There have been studies that suggest CYP 2E1 is also used in the metabolizing of kavalactones—kava compounds—metabolized by the same enzyme, or may have a similar enzymatic pathway. Then it is quite possible that when used in combination, the metabolic pathways become stressed and hepatotoxicity (toxic liver damage) may be more likely to occur.

Furthermore, kavalactones do temporarily alter the functioning of various liver enzymes, including gamma-glutamyl transferase and alkaline phosphatase. Some of the affected enzymes may be used during the metabolic processes of breaking down ethanol (alcohol). As a result, it is possible that enzymes

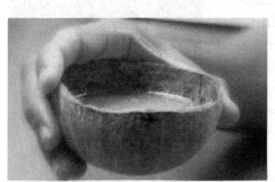

Sharing kava brew bonds friendships.

used in the metabolization of alcohol are temporarily affected while the liver processes kava kava. If this is the case, then it is likely that when kava kava is in the system, the liver may not be able to properly metabolize alcohol and could then experience hepatotoxicity if the substances are combined.

Camaraderie

The feelings of camaraderie that kava drinking evokes have made it a symbol for peace and friendship in many island nations of the Pacific. The atmosphere of the preparation sets the mood for the drinking. Kava preparation is the beginning of "Kava Time" and determines the quality of the drink that is being shared, enjoyed and appreciated.

A cup of kava before bed promotes sleep. A cup of kava brew is a good way to relax at the end of a hard day's work. Kava mixes well with cannabis, but alcohol and other CNS depressants should never be mixed with kava. Driving and operating dangerous machinery should be avoided.

Kava is a benign of sedative herb, causing neither addiction or dangerous physical effects. As with any powerful herb, it can be misused. Consciousness altering substances, like kava, should be used with wisdom, and moderation.

Generally speaking, a kava tea or traditonal prepared cold brew made with fresh root will have a higher concentraiton of active kavalactones than kava pills or capsules made from died material. The kind of kava supplemets you get from health food stores are usually made with older ground root and tend to be diminished in potency and effects. You are likely to get more potent and fresher kava ingredients from-venders specializing in kava and other herbs.

Kava Bars

Thousands of years before alcohol and coffee dominated the social scene, kava was the beverage of choice for every occasion in the-South Pacific Islands where kava was drunk in large quantities throughout the day. As kava has come into vogue, bars serving kava cocktails have been opening across America. Kava bars first opened in Florida and Hawaii beach communities and have spread into other regions. Some kava bars serve only traditional kava brews, while other bars serve non-noble kava varieties, or offer kava cocktails along with alcohol beverages.

House of Kava in Brooklyn is one of the first kava

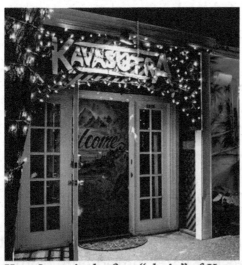

KavaSutra is the first "chain" of Kava Bars across the nation.

bars to open in New York City. About how the bar was received, co-founder Joyci Borovsky said, "Our first timers have all had very positive

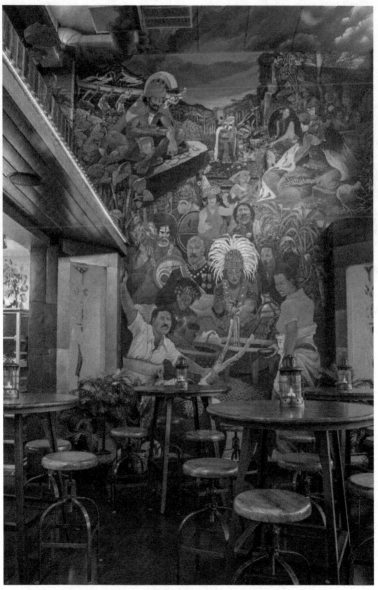

Root of Happiness in Davis, California.

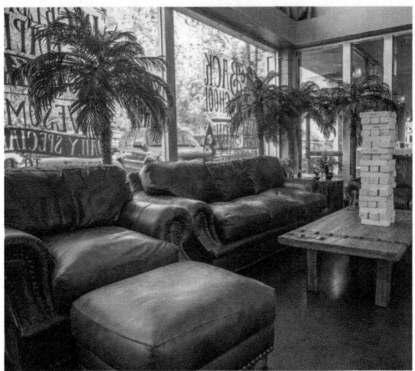

Root of Happiness is introducing kava by pulling from elements of Polynesian, Melanesian, and Micronesian Cultures for its richness of décor and ambiance.

experiences. People are very open to the idea of kava and once they try it they end up loving it. Kava itself mixed in with the environment at the bar makes for a relaxing, peaceful, and stress relieving experience". Patrons include office employees heading to work in the morning, developers and creative professionals. To adapt to local tastes, House of Kava offers kava cocktails with a chocolate flavor that is sweet with a hint of spice along with the traditional brew.

The positive physical and psychological effects of kava, combined with the environment at the bar, make for a relaxing, peaceful, and stress-relieving experience. Many claim that kava is a healthy alternative to alcohol for its

> **Ambiance is Central:**
>
> *KavaSutra Kava Bars have a relaxing, tranquil environment where you can come in, kick back, drink a kava shell, and relax within a non-judgmental and welcoming environment.*

ability to produce euphoria and relaxation without affecting mental clarity.

Kava bars, such as Kava Lounge, have opened across America in San Francisco, MeloMelo in Berkeley, and SquareRüt in Austin. KavaSutra—like KamaSutra, get it?—is a chain of kava bars with six locations, including Denver, New York City and four Florida cities. Root of Happiness, which offers wholesale and retail products online, is another emerging chain with bars in Davis and Rancho Cordova outside Sacramento, California.

Kava bars are a pleasant social environment somewhat like coffee houses with comfortable seating, relaxing lighting and the opportunity to strike up friendly conversations. Kava bartenders socialize with patrons while telling the history and positive effects of kava. They teach patrons to cheer "Bula!" when sharing drinks.

Bula Spirit

Bula, like Hawaiian *aloha*, is a Fijian word imbued with meanings depending on the situation. Pronounced as "boolah", it means "life" and is commonly used as a greeting, like *hello*. Saying *bula* expresses wishes for good health. The full saying is *"Ni sa bula vinaka"*—pronounced as "nee-sahm-bula-veenaka", which is similar to "wishing you happiness and good health." An appropriate response to bula in this context is *"Bula vinaka."*

Many kava bars greet guests by playing "Bula Malaya," a welcoming song expressing warmth and island hospitality. The word *bula* expresses feelings of affection and welcome called "Bula Spirit." "Bula Spirit" is a commitment to make an extra effort to ensure that the guest enjoys the very best in hospitality, warm thoughtful service and the kindness.

The Happiness Root

Kava is a wonderful social drink that makes patrons talkative, happy, and relaxed. Patrons sleep well after a night drinking kava. And, unlike after visiting a traditional alcohol bar, they have no unpleasant hangover or side effects in the morning.

The relaxation that accompanies drinking kava mimics the disinhibition brought about by alcohol and tension relieved with a few tokes of cannabis. The biggest difference is that Kava

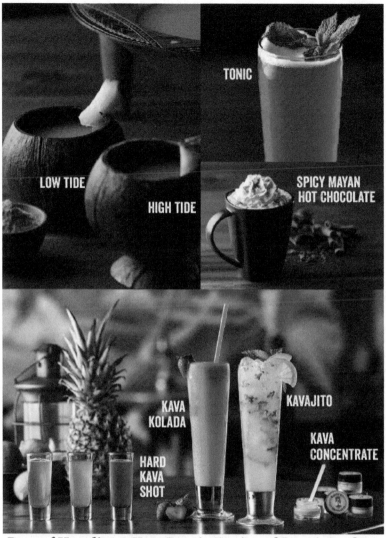

Root of Happliness Kava Bars in Davis and Ranco Cordova feature a fabulous array of Kava "potions".

doesn't alter mental clarity. Visiting a kava bar during the day is a bit like stopping off at a coffee house at lunch rather than a bar serving alcohol.

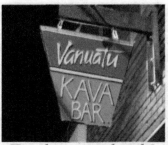

Kava bars are relaxed & friendly.

Many of the early kava bars revolved around words like *spirituality* and *ambiance*, and some even offered yoga practices, embracing the "be your best self" health trend that's popular. In the South Pacific the kava bar is the center of the community. It's the neighborhood watering hole where you go to see friends and drink a few rounds while catching up on local gossip.

Because kava makes folks feel relaxed and happy, it spurs conversation between strangers, making it easy to make friends. Kava bars are friendly and a place where it is acceptable for women to go to solo.

Kava Therapeutics

K ava root is an anesthetic with potency similar to that of cocaine and procaine. It numbs the tongue and the throat when drunk or taken orally as a liquid extract.

Traditional Therapeutic Uses

- Anxiety and depression
- Insomnia
- To relieve fatigue and to increase energy
- Genito-urinary tract disinfectant for urinary and reproductive organs infections
- Rheumatism
- Asthma
- For worms and parasites, a common problem in tropical climates
- For obesity
- Poultice for headaches
- Warm sweat inducing tea for the treatment of colds and fevers
- Topically for various skin diseases including fungal infections and leprosy

Urogenital Conditions

Kava is often used in the form of an alcoholic extract—a tincture—as an antiseptic remedy in the treatment of chronic irritation of the genito-urinary tract, especially that which is due to gonorrhea, and catarrh of the urethra and of the bladder. Chemicals in kava have a marked action in reducing the acidity of the urine and may be given with benefit in cases where there is an uric acid predisposition.

Marpmann demonstrated that the constituent kawain possesses bacteriological properties, especially for the gonococcus, but also for the coli bacillus. For these purposes, kava is usually mixed in the form of one part of the fluid-extract or dry extract made from the resin obtained from the crude herb, dissolved in four parts of

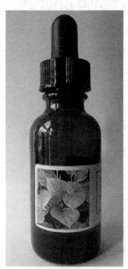

sandalwood oil, and given in capsules, but it is too irritating to be used for acute conditions.

On the South Pacific Islands, where kava was prepared by chewing, gonorrhea was rare, whereas in Tahiti—where little kava was consumed—cases of gonorrhea were very numerous. In the days when white men invaded the South Pacific Islands, where kava drinking

Kava tincture.

was the regular custom, many of the European sailors had gonorrhea; chronic cases of this disease, as well as

Kava is often used in an alcoholic extract in medicines, chiefly as an antiseptic remedy.

cases of chronic cystitis, are reported to have been cured within a few days by the natives with the help of kava.

Kava is useful in checking inflammatory discharge and in relieving pain of vaginitis, gonorrheal urethritis, metritis, salpingitis, enteritis and nocturnal incontinence of urine due to muscular weakness.

Since the discovery of the sulphonamidcs and penicillin, the importance of balsamic herbs—such as kava—in the treatment of venereal and other diseases has greatly declined. But the dual action—narcotic and antiseptic— of kava rootstock in the form of an emulsion makes it highly possible that the herb can be used successfully in a number gynecological, urological and other diseases; the herb certainly deserved to be tested clinically on a wide variety of diseases, seeing that the antibiotics and penicillin not infrequently cause considerable side-effects, and also because penicillin sometimes fails.

Dose

As a purely antiseptic remedy, kava is usually prescribed in the following daily doses:

Powdered root:

2 drams = 120 grains = about 8 gram.

Fluid-extract:

1 dram = 60 grains = about 4 grams.

Dry extract:

5-15 grains = 0.325-1 gram.

Divide into 3 or 4 portions and take after meals.

Other Conditions

Many drink kava to relieve headaches, restore vigor, promote urination, soothe unruly stomach, and to cure whooping cough and ease the symptoms of asthma. Topically, kava is useful in treating fungal infections and for soothing stings and skin irritations.

Kava has been used to treat bronchitis, diarrhea, gout, rheumatism, nephritic colic, dropsy, and colpitis. It is also used for attention deficit-hyperactivity disorder (ADHD), withdrawal from benzodiazepine drugs, epilepsy, psychosis, depression, migraines and other headaches, chronic fatigue syndrome (CFS), common cold and other respiratory tract infections, tuberculosis, muscle pain, and cancer prevention.

Habit Forming Potential

Habit forming is a risk of using of excessive doses of an emulsion, for intemperate potions of the beverage prepared by chewing can have a fatal effect. An emulsion might well be compared with the native beverage prepared by chewing, since saliva in the latter and sub-division of the rootstock do practically the same to the crude root as do water and oil in the process of intense emulsification through hygienic techniques.

The active principles dihydrokawain—marindinin—and dihydromethysticin can be liberated from the crude rootstock through a process of emulsification—chewing a modern technique—if chemically isolated—also need to be dispersed if a narcotic effect is aimed at. Wc learned too that a beverage prepared by maceration is merely a tonic, stimulant and antiseptic. The statement that the active principles arc supposed to be soluble in gastric juices, requires further investigation.

In homoeopathy, an extract of the rootstock, has been recommended in cases of cerebral congestion, fatigue and neuralgic headache. According to homoeopathic theory, homoeopathic doses have an effect different from those of allopathic doses.

Caution:

Never use kava when taking prescription drugs or using alcohol.

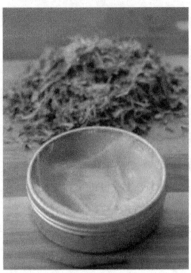

Kava salve can soothe sore
muscles.

Sore Muscles

Kava is an excellent analgesic and muscle relaxant, taking away the pain of an aching back or a sore neck. It has no side effects when taken in moderation, but if abused can cause health problems.

Summary

Kava rootstock used in the form of a maceration, taken internally, has merely a tonic, stimulant and antiseptic action. The crude root can exert its dual action— narcotic and antiseptic—only when made into the form of a suspension. Chemically isolated active principles (dihydrokaCain = marindinin, and dihydromethysticin) must be brought into the form of an emulsion to be physiologically active as a narcotic; they have perhaps an antibiotic effect, if not emulsified. It appears that isolation of the active principles is only possible in low yields and by tedious methods and that it is far better to use the crude drug in its entirety.

There is reason to believe that physicians can use the kava in the form of an emulsion for oral administration, among other ways, as an excellent tranquillizer, sedative and somnifacient medicine, in many cases in preference to morphine.

Soothing Anxiety

Drinking kava makes people feel happy and relaxed, while mental acuity remains intact, with no sense of hangover and rarely any irritability. Kava's therapeutic benefits stem from its influence on the limbic system, which is a set of primitive brain structures that control behavior and emotions.

Kava is one of the most powerful of all the herbal antispasmodics useful for relieving nervous tension throughout the mind and body. Kava is an anti-anxiety herb that will almost instantly dissipate effects of the many fears and apprehensions that are so much a part of the hectic modern lifestyle.

Clincial master herbalist Donnie

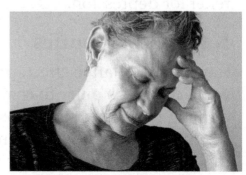

Many struggle with anxiety.

> *Kava offers a safe, effective alternative to prescription drugs for anxiety and insomnia and can provide relief for depression.*

Yance, MH. CN, notes that many people feel anxious when stressed, but for approximately 40 million Americans, anxiety is more than a passing emotion. Shortness of breath, racing heartbeat, dizziness, upset stomach, tension, irritability, sleep difficulties, memory problems, and feelings of dread are common daily experiences of people who suffer from chronic anxiety.

For those who consult a physician, the first suggestion is usually drugs: tranquilizers—benzodiazepines, often coupled with antidepressants, such as selective serotonin reuptake inhibitors (SSRIs). However, these medications come with a long list of unpleasant side effects, and have a significant risk of dependence. Kava offers a safe, effective alternative to prescription drugs for anxiety and insomnia, and can provide relief for depression.

Kava Therapeutics

Kava has a sedative effect, producing brainwave changes similar to changes that occur with calming medicines such as Valium. According to Michael Tierra, O.M.D., Founder of the American Herbalists Guild, kava has important therapeutic properties, including being a powerful herbal antispasmodic especially useful for relieving nervous tension and anxiety throughout the mind and body.

When drinking kava brew, feel-good vibes are sent to the brain through neurotransmission, which aid muscle relaxation, increase concentration, decreases insomnia, lower inhibitions and can also be suitable for pain such as back aches or hyperactivity in children. Many theorize that kava affects serotonin and dopamine neurotransmitters.

A 2003 study published in the *Canadian Medical Association Journal* reported that scientific evidence from randomized, placebo-controlled, double-blind studies have concluded that kava is an effective treatment for anxiety.

A randomized, placebo-controlled, double-blind study by Kinzler, Krömer and Lehmann showed that kava significantly reduced anxiety in humans. Two groups of 29 people with normal anxiety were treated for four weeks with three daily doses of 100 mg of kava rhizome extract or a placebo. After one week of treatment, subjects in the kava group had significantly lower anxiety levels compared with that of the placebo group, and the difference between

Kava is so effective at reducing anxiety it's been called "nature's Valium".

> *Traditionally people have dealt with these symptoms for anxiety by turning to alcohol and prescription drugs and sleep aids.*

the two groups increased during the course of the study. Over four weeks, kava extract progressively reduced anxiety compared with placebo in 60 patients with no reported adverse reactions.

A long 25-week, double-blind, placebo-controlled study of 101 patients with anxiety disorders conducted by Volz and Kieser found that Hamilton Anxiety Scale (HAMA) scores decreased faster with kava than with placebo.

Does Not Sedate the Mind

Kava does not interfere with mental sharpness because kava does not sedate the mind. A 2004 study found that 300 mg of kava may improve mood and cognitive performance. That is significant because some prescription drugs used to treat anxiety, such as benzodiazepines like Valium and alprazolam or Xanax, tend to decrease cognitive function.

While kava may be used instead of such prescription antianxiety drugs and tricyclic antidepressants, it should never be taken with prescription drugs. Likewise, drinking alcohol should be avoided.

How Kava Relieves Anxiety

Theory 1: Kavalactones clear the area around the receptor sites for a brain compound called gamma-amino butyric acid—GABA, so that more of the neutrotransmitters can connect to the receptors. The more GABA binds to receptors, the more relaxed we become.

Theory 2: Kava somehow acts on a part of the brain called the amygdala. The amygdala are two chickpea-sized lobes located in the limbic system of the brain. Amygdala are the parts of the brain that function improperly when anxiety hits. Neurotransmitters are out of balance in these tiny lobes during bouts of

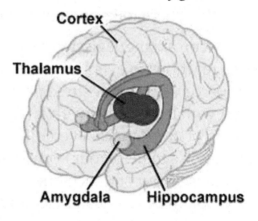

anxiety. The limbic system is the part of the brain that controls emotions, instinct, and basic body functions like heart rate, blood pressure, body temperature, blood sugar levels, sex drive, sleeping, waking and appitite.

But kava is also drunk to relieve headaches, to restore vigor in the face of general weakness, to promote urination, to soothe an unruly stomach, to cure whooping cough in children, and to ease the symptoms of asthma and tuberculosis. Topically, kava is useful to treat fungal infections and for soothing stings and skin inflammation.

Stress

Effects of stress and anxiety can include weakening immunity, nervousness, indigestions, difficulty concentrating, sleeplessness, chronic fatigue and an overall harassed feeling. It can blossom into panic attacks where folks are taken to the hospital.

Medical language stresses a series of physiological reactions to events. When we faced with real or perceived danger stress prepares our body to run with it or to deal with it. This sets off a whole chain of biochemical events, including surges of hormones to help your body defend itself. Muscles get tense, your stomach knots up, your heart races, your palms sweat—all reactions to prepare you to deal with a dangerous events. If stress goes on unrentlingly and is chronic. There can be trouble when all of these chemicals dumping into your body take it out of alignment and create conditions for disease and malfunction

Traditionally people have dealt with these symptoms for anxiety by turning to alcohol, prescription drugs, and sleep aids. According to the

National Foundation for Brain Research. Seventeen percent to 2twenty-three percent of adult
US women and eleven percent to seventeen
percent of US men suffer from anxiety disorder.
There is a well-established connection between
anxiety and depression. Not all depression is associated with anxiety, but anxiety is still a common symptom of depression, so that the lines
between the two conditions are blurred. The
drug of choice for depression is Prozac, which is
dispensed freely by physicians.

Part of the syndrome of depression or anxiety
is sleeplessness. It is estimated that 60 percent
of American adults ex-
perience some degree of
of occasional insomnia.
They may have trouble
falling asleep, or they
may wake up in the

*Scientists are still
uncovering exactly
how kava exerts its
sedative action.*

night and not be able to get back to sleep. Or
they may sleep fitfully, just being half asleep all
night long.

Constituients in kava are versatile and work in
different ways in the body. They can act directly on
muscles, interact with various brain chemicals and
influence part of the brain. Kava is a mild muscle
relaxing agent. When drinking kava, your limbs
might feel a little rubberly, perhaps tingly. Generally as muscles relax you experience a mellow
feeling.

Helps Generalized Anxiety Disorder

While kava has been used as an unregulated herbal treatment for generations because of its calming qualities, it has come to the attention of the medical community as a possible treatment for generalized anxiety disorder (GAD). For people with GAD, there are many treatment options. Most involve the assistance of a mental health professional, such as a counselor, psychiatrist, or psychologist, and the use of prescription drugs such as Prozac and Celexa.

For people who want to avoid taking anti-anxiety medications, lifestyle changes are usually suggested. Dietary and exercise changes can help decrease the anxiety. But anxiety isn't something a person can simply "think their way out of" or decide not to feel. Gen-

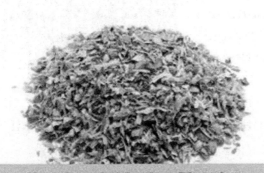

Kava Root For Anxiety Disorder

eralized anxiety disorder is a very real condition that needs to be addressed with the help of someone professionally trained to diagnose and treat it.

A number of clinical studies—though not all—have found kava to be effective in treating symptoms associated with anxiety. In a review of seven scientific studies, researchers concluded that a standardized kava extract was significantly more effective than placebo in treating anxiety. Another study found that kava substantially improved symptoms after only one week of treatment. According to another study, kava and diazepam—Valium—cause similar changes in brain wave activity, suggesting they may work in the same ways to calm the mind.

Dr. Jerome Sarris and colleagues at the University of Melbourne conducted a study with 37 people with generalized anxiety and varying levels of depression. In the first week, all participants took a placebo. In the second week, half the participants took kava tablets and the other half took placebo tablets. In the third week, the group that had taken kava tablets was switched to a placebo and the group that had taken a placebo switched to kava tablets. Participants were not aware whether they were taking a placebo or kava.

As measured by standardized anxiety and depression questionnaires, the participants reported much less anxiety when they were taking the kava than when they took placebo pills, Sarris says. Depression levels also dropped among many patients who reported depression and no serious side effects were associated with kava use. "What we can say is the evidence supports the use of this [formulation] for short periods for acute anxiety and stress," Sarris says.

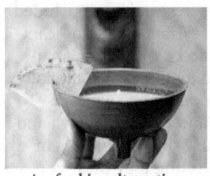

A refreshing alternative.

In 2013, research-ers at Rutgers and Adelphi Universities reviewed all the pub-lished research on nat-ural anxiety remedies. They concluded that kava is the most-stud-ied natural remedy for anxiety, and demonstrates the best results in clinical trials. A little later, a double-blind, pla-cebo-controlled study published in the *Journal of Clinical Psychopharmacology* confirmed the earlier reports of kava's clinical effectiveness for anxiety.

Alternative to Pharmecueticals

In another University of Melbourne project re-searchers studied kava as an alternative to phar-maceuticals. The study involved 75 participants who had been diagnosed with generalized anx-iety disorder, the most common anxiety condi-tion. Sarris and colleagues designed a six-week study to compare kava extract to placebo. For the first three weeks, they gave each participant either placebo or kava tablets twice per day.

The kava tablets consisted of a water-solu-ble extract of peeled kava root that included a total daily dose of 120 mg kavalactones, kava's primary active constituent. If the participants didn't experience any improvement after three weeks, their dose of placebo or kava was doubled so that the total daily dose of kavalactones was 240 mg.

Results showed a significant reduction in anxiety for the kava group compared to the placebo group at the end of the study. Participants diagnosed with moderate to severe generalized anxiety disorder had the greatest responses to kava's anxiety-reducing effects. In fact, by the end of the study, 26 percent of those in the Kava group had such large decreases in their anxiety symptoms that they were no longer classified as having an anxiety disorder, compared to only 6 percent in the placebo group. Interestingly, the researchers noted that kava increased women's sex drive compared to those in the placebo group, an effect that was likely due to lowered anxiety levels.

Kava was well-tolerated overall, and aside from more headaches reported in the kava group, results showed no considerable adverse reactions that could be attributed to Kava and no differences in signs of withdrawal or addiction between the kava and placebo groups.

Although the efficacy of kava is apparent, scientists are still uncovering exactly how kava exerts its sedative action. So far, researchers have found that kava affects gamma-amino-butyric acid—GABA—receptors in the brain; these receptors promote feelings of relaxation.

Other studies have shown that kava acts on the limbic system of the brain, which influences the emotions. Kava has also been found to block the uptake of noradrenaline, a hormone that triggers the physiological stress response.

How to Best Use Kava For Anxiety

University Health News Daily recommends that if you want to try kava as a natural remedy for anxiety, look for extracts that list the amount of kavalactones in milligrams per serving. They suggest taking the equivalent of 60 to 120 mg kavalactones twice per day, for a daily total of 120 to 240 mg kavalactones.

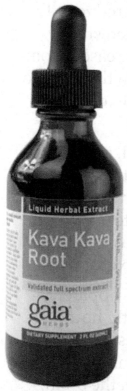

Kava does not alleviate anxiety immediately in everyone. While some people feel more relaxed after one dose, for others it can take as long as two months to experience the desired level of anxiety relief. Because kava generally causes drowsiness, it's recommended that it be taken it in the evening.

Note: Children under 18, women who are breast-feeding or nursing, and people on prescription medication should avoid kava and always consult with a medical professional before using it.

Kava Tincture.

Kava and Sleep

Because of its soothing, soporific effects, kava is used therapeutically by many to treat sleeplessness and anxiety. Michael J. Breus, Ph.D., a sleep specialist writing on WebMD, says that kava probably encourages sleep by reducing the anxiety and stress that is a common cause of sleeplessness.

Everyday stress, especially the inability to settle thoughts before bedtime, is a huge factor in sleeplessness. Kava offers a kind of "reset" button by helping to achieve a state of relaxed calm, making it that much easier to drift into restful sleep. Kava's mild analgesic and muscle relaxant properties help soothe mild aches and pains that can interfere with rest and help the body unwind physically before bed.

> *Kava is a first rate sedative producing a state of calm and promoting sleep.*

A double-blind placebo-controlled study by Saletu et al in 1989 found that doses of synthetic kavain between 200 and 600 mg "enhances brain activity that favors restorative sleep... EEG [electroencephalogram] activity showed that kavain increased the alpha-1, theta, and delta waves that are associated with sleep while decreasing beta waves, which are a sign of wakefulness". These effects increased as the dose of kavain was increased, so that "600mg of kavain produced sedation comparable to 30mg of clobazapam", a benzodiazepine drug used as a control.

As reported in the *Journal of Affect Disorders*, researcher Lehrl assessed the effects of kava extract WS 1490 on sleep disturbances associated with anxiety disorders. After four weeks of double-blind treatment, the assessment of quality of sleep and recuperative effect after sleep were statistically significant in comparison with placebo. Thus, a potential role for kava in improving sleep in patients with anxiety was suggested.

How to Use Kava as a Sleep Aid

Kava can be used in a number of different forms as an effective sleep aid. When taken for sleep problems, kava promotes deep sleep without affecting restful REM sleep. If you

Mixing, brewing, and straining the brew can be quite meditative.

want to take kava therapeutically for anxiety or sleep, make sure to follow the FDA's dosage guidelines of no more than 290 mg of kavalactones per day. Do

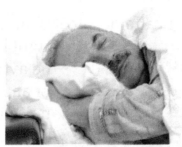

Kava promotes sound sleep.

this at least until you're more familiar with how kava affects you.

Most commonly, people consume a kava-based drink. Many enjoy the calming ritual of preparing kava before bedtime. Just as brewing a cup of hot tea or warm milk is relaxing, preparing and sipping a cup of kava before bed can put you into a mood to sleep. Mixing, brewing, and straining the brew can be quite meditative and an effective sleep ritual in itself. Nighttime rituals can markedly improve quality of sleep. Setting aside an hour or so of quiet time before bed allows the mind to unwind and let go of the thoughts of the day, which can otherwise disturb sleep.

Kava's effects are gradual in nature. When using kava you get a sleepy feeling without being "knocked out" and without becoming "dull" and unfocused. Instead, kava users report feeling alert and focused, able to think and remember clearly until drifting off into gentle slumber.

Other Sleep Aids

Intake of caffeine, alcohol and sugar, especially right before bed should be avoided. The amount of ambient light and noise in your bedroom should be reduced. Developing healthy sleep routines is very beneficial. These include ceasing the use of electronics two hours before sleep and making sure to eat the last meal about three hours before going to bed.

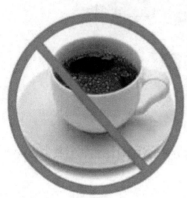

Don't Use Kava With Drugs

If you are using any prescription medication, make sure to talk to your prescribing doctor before using kava. Several adverse interactions with kava and drugs have been documented, both prescription and nonprescription—including, but not limited to, anticonvulsants, alcohol, anxiolytics or CNS depressants such as benzodiazepines, antipsychotics, levodopa, diuretics, and drugs metabolized by the liver.

Possible Interactions

The University of Maryland Medical Center advises to avoid using kava if you are being treated with a drug for a disease except with the supervision of your doctor. They caution to not take kava with prescription or over-the-counter medications.

Anticonvulsants — Kava may increase the effects of medications to treat seizures, such as phenytoin (Dilantin).

Anti-anxiety agents — Kava may increase the effects of CNS depressants such as benzodiazepines used for sleep disturbances or anxiety (particularly alprazolam or Xanax), and barbiturates (such as pentobarbital), which are used for sleep disorders and seizures. Benzodiazepines include:

- Alprazolam (Xanax)

- Diazepam (Valium)

- Lorazepam (Ativan)

- Triazolam (Halcion)

- Chlordiazepoxide (Librium)

Diuretics (water pills) – Diuretics help flush excess fluids from the body. Using kava with diuretics risks dehydration because kava makes the effects of them stronger.

Phenothiazine medications -- Drugs used to treat schizophrenia, including chlorpromazine (Thorazine); and promethazine (Phenergan), an antihistamine, should not be taken when using kava because it may increase the risk of side effects associated with these medications.

Levodopa – A chronic side effect of the drug, levodopa, that Parkinson's patients experience is the "on-off "phenomenon" of motor fluctuations where there will be periods of oscillations between "on" where the patient experiences symptomatic relief, and "off", where the therapeutic effect wears off early. There is evidence that when levodopa and kava are used together there is an increased frequency of this "on-off" phenomenon.

Medications metabolized by the liver — Kava may affect medications that are metabolized by the liver because it works on the liver. Again, consult your doctor about any medication you are using before taking kava.

Alcohol—Do not use alcohol and kava and together because risk of impairment and possible liver damage are greatly increased.

Avoid Using Kava
With These Drugs

Antianxiety Drugs

Atarax, Vistaril (hydroxyzine)
Ativan (lorazepam)
BuSpar (buspirone)
Centrax (prazepam)
Dalmane (flurazepam hudrochloride)
Doral (quazepam)
Equanil, Miltown (meprobamate)
Halcion (triazolam)
Klonopin (clonazepam)
Lectopam (bromazepam)
Loftran (ketazolam)
Librium, Libritabs (chlordiazepoxide)
Mogadon (nitrazepam)
Paxipam (halazepam)
Restoril (temazepam)
Serax (oxazepam)
Trancopal (chlormezanone)
Tranzene (clorazepate)
Valium, Vazepam (diazepam)

Antidepressant Drugs
Prozac (fluoxetine hydrochloride)
Effexor (venlafaxine hydrochloride)
Elavil, Endep (amitriptyline hydrochloride)
Asendin (amoxapine)
Anafranil (clomipramine hydrochloride)
Norpramin, Pertofrane (desipramine hydrochloride)
Adapink, Sinequan (doxepin hydrochloride)
Janimine, Tofranil (imipramine hydrochloride)
Aventyl, Pamelor (nortiptyline hydrochloride)
Vivactil (protriptyline hydrochloride)
Surmontil (trimipramine maleate)
Ludiomil (maprotiline hydrochloride)
Wellbutrin (bupropion)
Luvox (fluvoxamine maleate)
Serzone (paroxetine hydrochloride)
Paxil (paroxetine hydrochloride)
Zoloft (sertraline hydrochloride)
Desyrel (trazodone hydrochloride)
Versed (midazolam hydrochloride)
Xanax (alprazolam)

Any Monamine Oxidase Inhibitor

From Mindell, Earl, *All About Kava*. Avery, 1998.

14

Liver Toxicity Risk

There has been a concern about the safety of kava, particularly in regards to liver toxicity. Approximately one hundred people worldwide have been diagnosed with liver toxicity associated with kava use. In 2007, a safety panel of the World Health Organization (WHO) reported a possible link between kava use and seven deaths and 14 liver transplants, mostly in Europe.

These concerns came as a surprise to most users, given the fact that kava has been used for centuries by South Pacific Islanders without any ill-effect. The National Library of Medicine has stated "Based upon reported cases, the estimated frequency of clinically apparent liver injury due to kava is less than 1:1,000,000 daily doses."

Possible Hepatotoxicity

The National Institute of Diabetes and Digestive and Kidney Disease reported possible hepatotoxicity but the frequency of adverse liver reactions to kava is not known—although there seem to be convincing evidence of the possibility of hepatitis ending in fulminant hepatic failure, requiring liver transplantation, and even leading to death. Typical symptoms include fatigue, nausea, elevations in serum aminotransferase levels, and jaundice 2 to 24 weeks after starting use of kava.

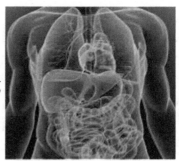

There is concern about possible damage to the liver.

In some cases, the pattern of enzyme elevations was hepatocellular, with elevations in serum aminotransferase and minimal increases in alkaline phosphatase levels. Sometimes there was immunoallergic hepatitis—rash, fever, eosinophilia, and recurrence on reexposure. The severity of liver injury ranges from transient and moderate enzyme elevations to symptomatic acute hepatitis to acute liver failure. In most instances, the liver injury subsides within 1 to 3 months of discontinuing the kava.

Possible Kava-Drug Interactions

The cause of hepatotoxicity is unclear. In vitro studies suggest that the kavalactones are not intrinsically cytotoxic, although other components of kava preparations may be. There may be herb-drug interaction.

The biggest problem is that the link between kava use and liver toxicity has not been established to a strong degree. Ernst reported in *British Journal of Clinical Pharmacology* in 2007 that the liver damage that patients suffered may have been the result of other drugs that were taken at the same time as the kava. In fact, in only fourteen of these cases was the liver toxicity s deemed to probably be a result of kava use. Putting this into perspective, Stevinson, Huntley and Ernst reported in *Drug Safety* that this shows there was one possible case of kava causing liver damage for every 100 million doses of kava that were sold—which is a pretty small risk, although it needs to be accounted for.

Only The Root Is Safe

The WHO report suggested that liver toxicity may be limited to kava formulations that used the whole kava plant, instead of just the root, or used acetone and ethanol to extract the active ingredient from the plant instead of water. Similarly, Richardson and Henderson suggested in the *British Journal of Clinical Pharmacology* that the kava used may have been incorrectly harvested and extracted.

Kava is a slow growing plant and because of its popularity at the time, it is believed that not enough kava was being produced. Only the root of the kava is safe to use. Suppliers may have included leaves and stems in their preparations.

The leaves and stems of a kava plant contain alkaloids that should not to be used in the kava extract.

By contrast, many studies have shown that kava use is safe. Sarris et al reported in *Phytotherapy Research* that they found no difference in liver functioning between the subjects who used kava and the subjects who did not. Additionally, there were no symptoms of withdrawal or addiction between the two groups, but there was a significant reduction in anxiety in the group taking

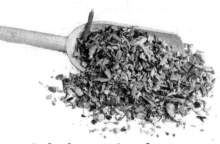

Only the root is safe to use.

kava. Clouatre examined reports of toxicity and reported in *Toxicology Letters* that, compared to other anti-anxiety drugs, the risk-to-benefit ratio of Kava use was very good.

Many professionals support kava's safety. Dr. Cott, the former Chief of the Psychopharmacology Research Program at the National Institute of Mental Health, reported that there is a greater chance of experiencing liver toxicity when taking acetaminophen than when using kava, and that anti-anxiety drugs and anti-depressants present a higher risk of liver toxicity than kava use.

Dr. Andrew Weil, of the Arizona Center for Integrative Medicine, agreed that kava use appeared safe for use, although he recommends using it no more than four weeks at a time without a break in use.

In conclusion, users need to take precautions that the kava being used is made from the root only and in the proper dosage. The risk of possibility liver toxicity is usually a result of improper kava extraction, mixing kava with hepatotoxic drugs or heavy alcohol use.

Bibliography

Ang-Lee M, Moss J, Yuan C. Herbal medicines and perioperative care. *JAMA*. 2001;286(2):208-216.

Anke J, Ramzan I. Pharmacokinetic and pharmacodynamic drug interactions with Kava (Piper methysticum Forst. f.). *J Ethnopharmacol*. 2004;93(2-3):153-60.

American Botanical Council. *American Botanical Council Announces New Safety Information on Kava*. 2001

Attele AS, Xie JT, Yuan CS. Treatment of insomnia: an alternative approach. *Altern Med Rev*. 2000;5(3):249-259.

Basch E, Ulbricht C, Hammerness P, et al. Kava monograph. *J Herbal Pharmacother*. 2002;2(4):65-91.

Baum SS, Hill R, Rommelspacher H. "Effect of kava extract and individual kavapyrones on neurotransmitter levels in the nucleus accumbens of rats". Prog. Neuropsychopharmacol. *Biol. Psychiatry. 1998, 22 (7): 1105–20.*

Beaubrun G, Gray GE. A review of herbal medicines for psychiatric disorders. *Psychiatr Serv*. 2000; 51(9):1130-1134.

Beckman SE, Sommi RW, Switzer J. Consumer use of St. John's wort: a survey on effectiveness, safety, and tolerability. *Pharmacotherapy*. 2000; 20(5):568-574.

Blumenthal M, Goldberg A, Brinckmann J, eds. *Herbal Medicine: Expanded Commission E Monographs*. Newton, MA: Integrative Medicine Communications; 2000: 221-225.

Boerner RJ, Klement S. Attenuation of neuroleptic-induced extrapyramidal side effects by Kava special extract WS 1490. *Wien Med Wochenschr*. 2004;154(21-22):508-510.

Boerner RJ, Sommer H, Berger W, et al. Kava-Kava extract LI 150 is as effective as Opipramol and Buspirone in Generalised Anxiety Disorder--an 8-week randomized, double-blind multi-centre clinical trial in 129 out-patients. *Phytomedicine*. 2003;10 Suppl 4:38-49.

Breus, Michael J. "Kava For Sleep? Why It Continues to Be a Mystery". *Huffington Post*. August 20th, 2011.

Cagnacci A, Arangino S, Renzi A, et al. Kava-Kava administration reduces anxiety in perimenopausal women. *Maturitas*. 2003;44(2):103-109.

Cairney S, Clough AR, Mruff P, Collie A. Currie BJ, Currie J. Saccade and Cognitive Function in Chronic Kava Users. *Neuropsychopharmacology, 2003, 28 (2): 389-96.*

Christi SU, Seifert A, Seeler D, Toxic hepatitis after consumption of traditional kava preparation. *J. Travel Med.* 2009, Jan-Feb: 16(1): 55-56.

Clouatre, D. L., Kava Kava: Examining New Reports of Toxicity. *Toxicology Letters*, 2004 150(1), 85-96.

Connor KM, Payne V, Davidson JR. Kava in generalized anxiety disorder: three placebo-controlled trials. *Int Clin Psychopharmacol*. 2006; 21(5):249-253.

Cropley M, Cave Z, Ellis J, et al. Effect of Kava and Valerian on human physiological and psychological responses to mental stress assessed under laboratory conditions. *Phytother Res*. 2002; 16(1):23-27.

Dasgupta, Amitava, Hammett-Stabler, Catherine A., *Herbal Supplements: Efficacy, Toxicity, Interactions with Western Drugs, and Effects on Clinical Laboratory Tests. John Wiley & Sons. March 2011, pp. 57*

De Smet PA. Safety concerns about kava not unique. *Lancet* 2002; 360(9342):1336.

Dinh LD, Simmen U, Bueter KB, Bueter B, Lundstrom K, Schaffner W. Interaction of various Piper methysticum cultivars with CNS receptors in vitro. *Planta 2001, Med.* **67** (4): 306–11.

Ernst, E. A re-evaluation of kava (*Piper methysticum*). *British Journal of Clinical Pharmacology,* 2007, 64(4), 415–417.

Ernst E. Safety concerns about kava. *Lancet* 2002; 359(9320):1865.

Ernst E. The risk-benefit profile of commonly used herbal therapies: Ginkgo, St. John's Wort, Ginseng, Echinacea, Saw Palmetto, and Kava. *Ann Intern Med.* 2002;136(1):42-53.

Escher M, Desmeules J, Giostra E, et al. Hepatitis associated with kava, a herbal remedy for anxiety. *BMJ.* 2001;322:139.

Fetrow CW, Avila JR. *Professional's Handbook of Complementary & Alternative Medicines .* 3rd ed. Philadelphia, PA: Lippincott Williams & Wilkins; 2004:472-477.

Freeman LW. *Mosby's Complementary & Alternative Medicine: A Research-Based Approach.* 3rd ed. St. Louis, MO: Mosby Elsevier; 2009:431-434.

Fu PP, Xia Q, Guo L, Yu H, Chan PC. Toxicity of kava kava. *J Environ Sci Health C Environ Carcinog Ecotoxicol Rev.* 2008 Jan-Mar;26(1):89-112. Review.

Garrett KM, Basmadjian G, Khan IA, Schaneberg BT, Seale T.W. Extracts of kava (Piper methysticum) induce acute anxiolytic-like behavioral changes in mice. *Psychopharmacology (Berl.).2003,* **170** *(1): 33–41.*

Gastpar M, Klimm HD. Treatment of anxiety, tension and restlessness states with Kava special extract WS 1490 in general practice: a randomized placebo-controlled double-blind multicenter trial. *Phytomedicine* 2003;10(8):631-639.

Gyllenhaal C, Merritt SL, Peterson SD, et al. Efficacy and safety of herbal stimulants and sedatives in sleep disorders. *Sleep Med Rev.* 2000;4(2):1-24.

Jamieson, D.D., Duffield, P.H., Positive interactions of ethanol and kava resin in mice. *Clinical and Experimental Pharmacology and Physiology*, 17, 509–51.

Jorm AF, Christensen H, Griffiths KM, Parslow RA, Rodgers B, Blewitt KA. Effectiveness of complementary and self-help treatments for anxiety disorders. *Med J Aust*. 2004;181(suppl 7):S29-S46

Kinzler E, Krömer J, Lehmann E. Effect of a special kava extract in patients with anxiety-, tension-, and excitation states of non-psychotic genesis. Double blind study with placebos over 4 weeks [in German]. *Arzneimittelforschung*. 1991;41(6):584-588.

LaValle JB, Krinsky DL, Hawkins EB, et al. *Natural Therapeutics Pocket Guide*. Hudson, OH:LexiComp; 2000: 466-467.

Lehrl S. Clinical efficacy of kava extract WS 1490 in sleep disturbances associated with anxiety disorders. Results of a multicenter, randomized, placebo-controlled, double-blind clinical trial. *J Affect Disord* 2004;78(2):101-110.

Ligresti A, Villano R, Allarà M, Ujváry I, Di Marzo V. Kavalactones and the endocannabinoid system: the plant-derived yangonin is a novel CB1 receptor ligand. *Pharmacol. Res.*2012, *66 (2): 163–9.*

Li XZ, Ramzan I. Role of ethanol in kava hepatotoxicity. *Phytother Res*. 2010;24(4):475-480.

Maneze D, Speizer A, Dalton N, Dennis S. A descriptive study of kava use among Tongan men in Macarthur, Sydney South West. *Aust N Z J Public Health*. 2008 Aug;32(4):314-316.

Olsen LR, Grillo MP, Skonberg C. Constituents in kava extracts potentially involved in hepatotoxicity: a review. *Chem. Res. Toxicol. 2011, 24 (7): 992–1002.*

Pittler MH, Ernst E. Kava extract for treating anxiety. *Cochrane Database Syst Rev*. 2002;(2):CD003383.

Rakel: *Integrative Medicine, 3rd ed.* Philadelphia, PA: Saunders, 2012.

Richardson, W. N., & Henderson, L. The safety of kava—a regulatory perspective. *British Journal of Clinical Pharmacology,* 2007, 64(4), 418–420.

Robbers JE, Tyler VE. *Tyler's Herbs of Choice: The Therapeutic Use of Phytomedicinals* . New York, NY: Haworth Herbal Press; 1999:157-159.

Rotblatt M, Ziment I. *Evidence-Based Herbal Medicine.* Philadelphia, PA: Hanley & Belfus, Inc; 2002:245-248.

Saletu, B., Grünberger, J., and Linzmayer, L. (1989). EEG-brain mapping, psychometric and psychophysiological studies on central effects of kavain–A kava plant derivative. *Human Psychopharmacology* 1989, 4: 169-190.

Sarris J, LaPorte E, Schweitzer I. Kava: a comprehensive review of efficacy, safety, and psychopharmacology. *Aust N Z J Psychiatry.*2011, *45 (1): 27–35.*

Sarris J, Kavanagh DJ, Deed G, Bone KM. St. John's Wort and Kava in treating major depressive disorder with comorbid anxiety: a randomised double-blind placebo-controlled pilot trial. *Hum Psychopharmacol.* 2009 Jan;24(1):41-48.

Sarris, J., Stough, C., Teschke, R., Wahid, Z. T., Bousman, C. A., Murray, G., Savage, K. M., Mouatt, P., Ng, C., & Schweitzer, I., Kava for the Treatment of Generalized Anxiety Disorder RCT: Analysis of Adverse Reactions, Liver Function, Addiction, and Sexual Effects. *Phytotherapy Research.* 2013

Singh YN, Singh NN. Therapeutic potential of kava in the treatment of anxiety disorders. *CNS Drugs.* 2002, 16 (11): 731-43.

Steiner GG. The correlation between cancer incidence and kava consumption. *Hawaii Med J* . 2000;59(11):420-422.

Stevinson, C., Huntley, A., & Ernst, E. (2002). A systematic review of the safety of kava extract in the treatment of anxiety. *Drug Safety*, 25, 251–61.

Teschke R, Gaus W, Loew D. Kava extracts: safety and risks including rare hepatotoxicity. *Phytomedicine.* 2003;10(5):440-446.

Teschke R, Sarris J, Lebot V. Contaminant hepatotoxins as culprits for kava hepatotoxicity--fact or fiction? *Phytother Res.* 2013; 27(3):472-474.

Teschke R, Schwarzenboeck A, Hennermann KH. Kava hepatotoxicity: a clinical survey and critical analysis of 26 suspected cases. *Eur J Gastroenterol Hepatol.* 2008 Dec;20(12):1182-1193.

Thompson R, Ruch W, Hasenohrl RU. Enhanced cognitive performance and cheerful mood by standardized extracts of Piper methysticum (Kava-kava). *Hum Psychopharmacol.* 2004;19(4):243-250.

van der Watt G, Laugharne J, Janca A. Complementary and alternative medicine in the treatment of anxiety and depression. *Curr Opin Psychiatry.* 2008 Jan;21(1):37-42. Review.

Volz HP, Kieser M. Kava-kava extract WS 1490 versus placebo in anxiety disorders—a randomized placebo-controlled 25-week outpatient trial. *Pharmacopsychiatry* . 1997;30(1):1-5.

Wheatley D. Kava and valerian in the treatment of stress-induced insomnia. *PhytotherRes.* 2001;15(6):549-551.

Witte S, Loew D, Gaus W. Meta-analysis of the efficacy of the acetonic kava-kava extract WS1490 in patients with non-psychotic anxiety disorders. *Phytother Res.* 2005;19(3):183-188.

Beverly A. Potter, PhD ("Docpotter") has created derivatives from many Works of Great Masters, helping their influence to be available and live on. Docpotter is based in Oakland, California. Her website—docpotter. com—is packed with useful information. *Please visit.*

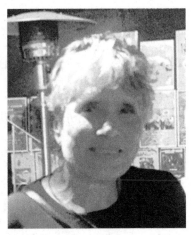

Docpotter

Other Derivatives By Docpotter

Timothy Leary

Your Brain Is God

Change Your Brain

Start Your Own Religion

CyberPunks; CyberFreedom

Search for the True Aphrodisiac

Alternatives to Involuntary Death

The Fugitive Philosopher

The Politics of Self-Determination

Politics of Psycho-Pharmacology

Evolutionary Agents

Musing on Human Metamorphsis

John C. Lilly

The Quiet Center

Programming the Human BioComputer

The Steersman:
Metabelif & Self-Navigation

John W. Aiken

Explorations in Awareness:
Finding God by Mediating with Entheogens

Sir John Lubbock

Simple Pleasures:
Tuning into NOW

Florence Sovel Shinn

Spiritual Secrets for Playing the Game of Life

Principis Discordia

Discordia:
Hail Eris Goddess of Chaos and Confusion

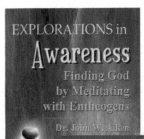

RONIN

Books for Independent Minds

Bookstores:
Order from PGW

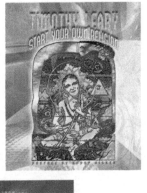

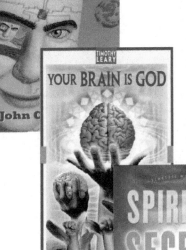

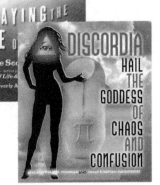

Use isbn to order
RONIN books
from any book-
store, Amazon, or
other online outlets.

CPSIA information can be obtained
at www.ICGtesting.com
Printed in the USA
LVOW05s0856270917
550237LV00004B/11/P